Biomedical Library

Queen's University Belfast

Tel: 028 9097 2710

E-mail: biomed.info@qub.ac.uk

For due dates and renewals:

QUB borrowers see 'MY ACCOUNT' at

http://library.qub.ac.uk/qcat

or go to the Library Home Page

HPSS borrowers see 'MY ACCOUNT' at

www.honni.qub.ac.uk/qcat

Springer

London
Berlin
Heidelberg
New York
Barcelona
Budapest
Hong Kong
Milan
Paris
Santa Clara
Singapore
Tokyo

P. Geusens (Ed.)

Osteoporosis in Clinical Practice

A Practical Guide for Diagnosis and Treatment

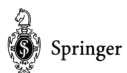

Springer

Professor P. Geusens
Clinical Research Center for Bone and Joint Diseases,
Dr L Willems-Instituut, Universitaire Campus, Buildings A and C,
B-3590 Diepenbeek, Belgium

Front cover picture by Dirk Boulanger

ISBN 3-540-76223-X Springer-Verlag Berlin Heidelberg New York

British Library Cataloguing in Publication Data
Osteoporosis in clinical practice : a practical guide for diagnosis and treatment
  1.Osteoporosis - Diagnosis 2.Osteoporosis - Treatment
  I.Geusens, P.
  616.7'16
  ISBN 354076223X

Library of Congress Cataloging-in-Publication Data
Osteoporosis in clinical practice : a practical guide for diagnosis
  and treatment / P. Geusens (ed.).
     p.   cm.
  Includes bibliographical references and index.
  1. Osteoporosis. 2. Physicians (General practice) I. Geusens, Piet.
  [DNLM: 1. Osteoporosis- -diagnosis. 2. Osteoporosis- -therapy.
  3. Diagnosis, Differential. WE 250 0851255 1998]
  RC931.07743 1998
  616.7'16- -dc21
  DNLM/DLC
  for Library of Congress   97-41383

Typeset by: Christopher Greenwell
Printed and bound by Bell and Bain Ltd, Glasgow, Scotland
28/3830-543210 Printed on acid-free paper

Foreword

Robert Lindsay

The field of osteoporosis has advanced significantly over the past several years. Only ten years ago many individuals, physicians and scientists considered the diagnosis of osteoporosis only when patients presented with fractures. We now consider fractures to be the clinical sequelae of the underlying disease that is defined as osteoporosis. This emphasizes the importance of the skeletal changes in the pathogenesis of the fractures that occur, while allowing clinical recognition of the other processes that lead to increased fracture risk in the aging population. Thus, the underlying skeletal disease is now defined as follows:

> *"Osteoporosis is a systemic skeletal disease characterized by low bone mass and micro-architectural deterioration of bone tissue, with a consequent increase in bone fragility and susceptibility to fracture risk."*

That definition, which clearly describes the pathophysiology of the disease is, however, less useful to the primary care physician who has to deal in a pragmatic fashion with patients who might be at risk of osteoporosis, or who already have the disease.

This volume addresses that issue. The editor, Dr. Piet Geusens, who is a world renowned expert in this disease, has assembled an impressive group of physicians and scientists to address the various aspects of this disease important in daily clinical practice.

It has been suggested that the average primary care physician will see two or more patients with osteoporosis every single day in practice, but recognize less than 10% of affected individuals, while treating only a fraction of those recognized. The redefinition of osteoporosis in terms of bone density, gives clinicians a tool to identify asymptomatic patients. Bone density predicts the risk of fractures. Consequently, a clear definition of who to measure, what test to use, and when (and how frequently) to order the test is fundamental to the prevention of osteoporotic fractures. In many respects, clinical practice in this area equates to the management of hypertension of cholesterol. By and large physicians are unaware of these tests, cannot easily interpret the results, and have not had clear guidance on when intervention is appropriate. A clear text providing this information is a timely addition to the primary care physicians' bookshelves, from which it should frequently be consulted.

Several approaches are available for both prevention and treatment of osteoporosis. Thus, on identification of high risk patients or those who already have fractures, physicians have the capacity to intervene with effective therapies.

Because of the overall impact of the disease, a significant research effort within the pharmaceutical industry is currently directed toward new therapeutic approaches, which physicians may have available in the future. However, in order to make best use of these new approaches, physicians need to increase their understanding of the disease and its current diagnosis and management in preparation for the increased choices of the future. It is clear that industry tactics are aimed at direct to consumer advertising, and consequently patients will be coming to physicians increasingly frequently with questions, and demands, relating to osteoporosis, its diagnosis and treatment. This clear and concise text will allow the interested physician, both specialist and primary care, to accomplish that.

Preface

Piet Geusens

I wait for the doctor with pains in my back ... When will he come ? ...
He will tell he had first to cure the fractured leg of Aesculapius and the fractured
arm of Apollo
Plautus, Menaechmi

It is part of the cure to wish to be cured
Seneca, Hippolytus

Science has a human and thus personal face. Especially when clinical scientists express their view in a concise form, to convince their audience about the scientific basis of clinical practice.

Osteoporosis is an example of a disease that has evolved from an inevitable sequence of events towards a clinical disease that can now be diagnosed and treated.

In this book, we have brought together scientists, who have devoted much of their time to unravel the backgrounds of such a frequently occuring disease as osteoporosis. The aim of their condensed contributions is to bring the progressing knowledge on osteoporosis within the reach of the busy practitioner in the first and second line of patient care.

Some overlap and difference in opinion between the chapters was inevitable. However, this can be informative too, since each chapter was conceived to answer specific questions that arise in daily clinical practice, when confronted with osteoporosis in an individual patient. In the final chapters, authors try to look into the future, as it is highly conceivable that new approaches for the diagnosis and treatment of osteoporosis will emerge within the next few years.

Acknowledgements
We thank Dr. M.-P. Jacobs, Dr. J. Vanhoof and Dr. K. Declerck for critical reading of the manuscript and P. Daniëls for administrative assistance.

Contents

Contributors

Glen M. Blake
Department of Nuclear Medicine, Guy's Hospital,
St Thomas Street, London SE1 9RT, UK

Jean-Jacques Body
Unit Endocrinology, Institut Jules Bordet,
1. Rue Heger Bordet, 1000 Brussels, Belgium

Henry G. Bone
Bone and Mineral Clinic P.C., 22201 Moross Road, Suite 260,
Detroit, Michigan MI 48236, USA

Steven Boonen
Department of Internal Medicine, Division of Geriatric Medicine,
University Hospitals, Brusselsstraat 69, 3000 Leuven ,Belgium.

Roger Bouillon
Onderwijs en Navorsing, LEGENDO,
U.Z. Gasthuisberg, Herestraat 49, 3000 Leuven, Belgium

Peter Burckhardt
Department of Medicine, CHUV-University Hospital,
1011 Lausanne, Switzerland

Jan Dequeker
Artritis/Met. Bone Research Unit, K.U. Leuven,
U.Z. Pellenberg, Welgelverd 1, 3212 Pellenberg, Belgium

Marie-Christine de Vernejoul
Inserm Unité de Recherche 349, Centre Viggo Petersen,
Hôpital Lariboisière, 6, rue Guy Patin, 75010 Paris, France

Linda Edwards
National Osteoporosis Society, P.O. Box 10,
Radstock, Bath BA3 3YB, UK

John Eisman
Bone and Mineral Research Program, Garvin Institute of Medical Research,
Prince of Wales Hospital, High Street, Randwick, Sydney NSW 2031, Australia

Ignac Fogelman
Department of Nuclear Medicine, Guy's Hospital,
St Thomas Street, London SE1 9RT, UK

Carlo Gennari
Institute of Internal Medicine and Medical Pathology, University of Siena,
Viale Bracci, Siena 53100, Italy

Piet Geusens
Clinical Research Center for Bone and Joint Diseases, Dr. L. Willems-Instituut,
Limburgs Universitair Centrum, Universitaire Campus, 3590 Diepenbeek, Belgium

Robert P. Heaney
John A. Creighton University, 2500 California Plaza,
Omaha, Nebraska NB 68178, USA

Klaus Hindso
Department of Orthopaedic Surgery, Bispebjerg Hvidovre Hospital,
University of Copenhagen, Bispebjerg Bakke 23, DK 2400 Copenhagen NV, Denmark

Olof Johnell
Department of Orthopaedic Surgery, Malmö University Hospital,
S 20502 Malmö, Sweden

Richard W. Keen
Twin and Osteoporosis Research Unit, St Thomas's Hospital,
Lambeth Palace Road, London SE1 7EH, UK

Michael Kleerekoper
Division of Endocrinology, Department of Internal Medicine, UHC-4H,
4201 St Antoine, Detroit, Michigan MI48201, USA

Robert Lindsay
Regional Bone Center, Helen Hayes Hospital, Route 9W,
West Haverstraw, New York NY 10993, USA

Jes B. Lauritzen
Department of Orthopaedic Surgery, Bispebjerg Hvidovre Hospital,
University of Copenhagen, Bispebjerg Bakke 23, DK 2400 Copenhagen NV, Denmark

Anthony R. Lyons
Department of Orthopaedic and Accident Surgery, C Floor, West Block,
University Hospital, Queen's Medical Centre, Nottingham NG7 2UH, UK

Nikolai A. Manassiev
Wynn Division of Metabolic Medicine, Imperial college School of Medicine,
National Heart and Lung Institute, 21 Wellington Road, London NW8 9SQ, UK

Robert Marcus
Aging Study Unit, Education and Clinical Center, Department of Veterans Affairs,
Medical Center, Stanford University, 3810 Miranda Avenue (182-B),
Palo Alto, California CA 94304, USA

Michael R. McClung
Oregon Osteoporosis Center, 5050 NE Hoyt, Suite 651,
Portland, Oregon OR 97213, USA

L. Joseph Melton III
Department of Health Sciences Research, Mayo Clinic, 200 First Street SW,
Rochester, Minnesota MN 55905, USA

Helmut W. Minne
Clinic Der Furstenhof, Clinic for Metabolic Bone Disease,
P.O. Box 1660, D 31798 Bad Pyrmont, Germany

Lis Mosekilde
Department of Cell Biology, Institute of Anatomy,
University of Aarhus, DK 8000 Aarhus C, Denmark

Vasi Naganathan
Department of Rheumatology, University of Sydney, Royal North Shore Hospital,
St Leonard's, Sydney, NSW 2065, Australia

Dorothy A. Nelson
Division of Endocrinology, Department of Internal Medicine, UHC-4H,
4201 St Antoine, Detroit, Michigan MI48201, USA

Karl J. Obrant
Department of Orthopaedic Surgery, Malmö University Hospital,
S 20502 Malmö, Sweden

Aurelio Rapado
Medicine Department Metabolic Unit, Fundacion Jiminez Diaz,
Avenida Reyes Catolicos 2, Madrid 28040, Spain

Ian R. Reid
Department of Medicine, University of Auckland,
Private Bag 92019, Auckland, New Zealand

Philip D. Ross
Hawaii Osteoporosis Foundation, 401 Kamakee Street, Second Floor,
Honolulu, Hawaii HI 96814-4224, USA

Rosemary Rowe
National Osteoporosis Society, P.O. Box 10,
Radstock, Bath BA3 3YB, UK

Philip N. Sambrook
Department of Rheumatology, University of Sydney, Royal North Shore Hospital,
St Leonard's, Sydney, NSW 2065, Australia

Maren G. Scholz
Clinic Der Furstenhof, Clinic for Metabolic Bone Disease,
P.O. Box 1660, D 31798 Bad Pyrmont, Germany

Ego Seeman
Department of Endocrinology, University of Melbourne, Austin Medical Center,
Heidelberg, Melbourne 3084, Australia

Mehrsheed Sinaki
Physical Medicine and Rehabilitation, Mayo Clinic, 200 First Street SW,
Rochester, Minnesota MN 55905, USA

Charles W. Slemenda[†]
Division of Biostatistics, University of Indiana School of Medicine,
RR 135, 702 Barnhill Drive, Riley Res. Wing, Indianapolis IN 46202-5200, USA

Tim D. Spector
Twin and Osteoporosis Research Unit, St Thomas's Hospital,
Lambeth Palace Road, London SE1 7EH, UK

John Stevenson
Wynn Division of Metabolic Medicine, Imperial college School of Medicine,
National Heart and Lung Institute, 21 Wellington Road, London NW8 9SQ, UK

Dirk Vanderschuren
Onderwijs en Navorsing, LEGENDO,
U.Z. Gasthuisberg, Herestraat 49, 3000 Leuven, Belgium

Chris White
Bone and Mineral Research Program, Garvin Institute of Medical Research,
St Vincent's Hospital, 384 Victoria Street, Darlinghurst, Sydney NSW 2010, Australia

In Memoriam

Charles Slemenda, Dr. P.H. suddenly collapsed and died on July 17th, 1997. Dr. Slemenda's principle interest was in osteoporosis where he made major contributions to the understanding of the disease. He had studied factors important in the development of peak bone mass, including genetics and nutrition. He had also studied variables important in loss of bone, such as changes in hormone concentrations.

In his short career he published over 75 papers, spoke at many national and international symposia, and served on a number of review panels.

Charles Slemenda will be remembered for his keen intellect, his honesty and dedication to his profession, his warm sense of humor, and his love for family and friends.

C. Conrad Johnston, Jr., M.D.

Indiana University, September 1997

1

Bone Structure and Function

Marie-Christine de Vernejoul

Bone consists of an abundantly calcified extracellular matrix. This tissue serves three functions: mechanical, protective for the vital organs and metabolic as a reserve of ions especially calcium and phosphate. Bone tissue undergoes continuous renewal in order to maintain the mechanical competence of the bone matrix. This is performed by two cells: osteoclasts which resorb the calcified matrix and osteoblasts that synthesize new bone matrix.

Bone Matrix

95% of the bone matrix is made of collagen I, the only collagen present in bone. The remaining part of the bone matrix includes proteoglycans. They might have a role in mineralization, but they also bind several growth factors (decorin binds transforming growth factor beta (TGF-β) and heparan sulfate binds fibroblast growth factor (FGF)). The non-collagenous proteins of bone are synthesized by the osteoblasts. Osteocalcin is the most abundant one and is specific for bone. Its function is not yet clear. The other non-collagenous proteins of bone, osteopontin, bone sialoprotein, and thrombospondin have an amino acid sequence (R-G-D) which mediates the attachment of the cells to the bone matrix and are involved in bone cells attachment and differentiation.

Bone matrix is the most abundant reservoir of the organism for growth factors. TGF-β and the other members of this family of growth factors, the bone morphogenetic proteins (BMP) are trapped in a latent form. The insulin-like growth factors (IGF-I and IGF-II) are bound to their binding proteins. Furthermore, the FGF is also present in the bone matrix. These growth factors are secreted by the osteoblasts and are also able to stimulate osteoblast recruitment and matrix synthesis.

Bone Cells and Bone Remodeling   *Bone Cell Biology*

Osteoclasts are highly specialized cells uniquely localized on endostal bone surfaces (Figure 1.1). Their origin is hematopoietic and they share a common precursor with the monocyte-macrophage. They are large polarized multinucleated cells with an average of 10 to 20 nuclei. Osteoclasts have a specialized cell membrane with folds and invagination at the interface with bone surface, called "ruffled border". In order to resorb the mineralized bone matrix, osteoclasts produce proteolytic enzymes and hydrogen ions in the

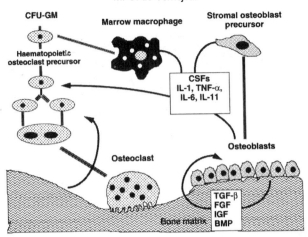

Figure 1.1. Bone cells and bone remodeling.

microcompartment localized between the ruffled border and bone. Among the enzymatic equipment of the osteoclasts aimed at degrading the bone matrix, the tartrate-resistant acid phosphatase is quite specific. The osteoclasts produce also enzymes, such as cathepsin-K able to degrade collagen. They are active at the low pH found in the resorption microcompartment. The acidification of the mineralized matrix depends on proton production by carbonic anhydrase-II, which deficiency induces the lack of bone resorption and osteosclerosis, and proton excretion by a proton pomp, of the vacuolar type, located at the ruffled border. The osteoclasts are attached to the bone matrix during the resorbing process by integrins, of which the vitronectin receptor is the most important one. It has been shown that inhibiting this protein impairs bone resorption. Osteoclasts have receptors for calcitonin, which induce retraction of the cell from the bone matrix and therefore a transient cessation of bone resorption.

Osteogenesis starts by recruitment and proliferation of pre-osteoblastic cells from a stem cell, progressive differentiation of these cells in **osteoblasts** and bone extracellular matrix synthesis. In the long bone the stem cell of osteoblast is present in the medullar stroma. The medullar stromal stem cell can give rise to adipocyte mesenchymal or chondroblast cells after induction by hormonal or local factors. Differentiation of osteoblasts is a complex issue. Initially, local mitogenic factors induce cell multiplication. During this phase of active proliferation cells express early genes such as oncogen c-fos and myc and histone H4. Phosphatase activity, an early marker of osteoblast function, appears also in this phase. After the proliferation phase, the osteoblasts express type I collagen, followed by osteocalcin and bone sialoprotein-I. Differentiating osteoblasts are attracted by chemotactism towards pre-existing bone matrix by growth factors and proteins of the matrix. Osteoblasts adhere to the matrix, polarize and secrete a new matrix. It is also believed that osteoblasts are directly involved in the mineralization of this matrix by budding from their cytoplasmic membrane of vesicules rich in alkaline phosphatases. Osteoblasts actively secrete all the growth

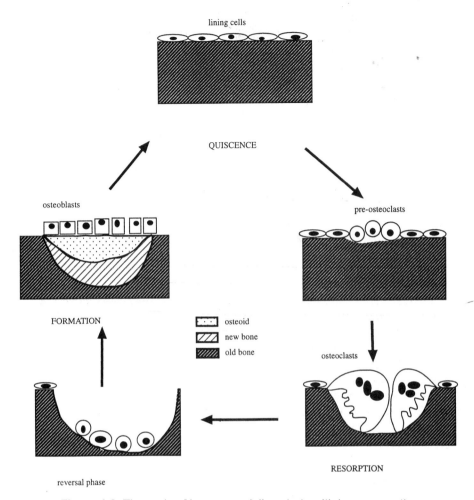

Figure 1.2. The cycle of bone remodeling starts with bone resorption and is followed by bone formation.

factors which will be trapped in the matrix. Also, they synthesize cytokines, mainly Interleukine-6 (IL-6), and the hematopoietic growth factor, Macrophage Colony Stimulating Factor (M-CSF) which might be responsible for osteoclast recruitment. Contrarily to the osteoclasts, the osteoblasts have receptors for several hormones including parathormone and estrogens and have a pivotal role in the response of the osteoclast to these hormones.

Bone remodeling is a process allowing renewal of bone matrix (Figure 1.2). The cycle of bone remodeling lasts approximately 3 months in adult human bone and about 1 million bone remodeling units are present in the human skeleton and are activated sequentially. The start of the remodeling sequence is the activation phase which corresponds to osteoclast differentiation. *In vitro* studies showed that soluble factors released by osteoblasts are required for this phase. These factors include the M-CSF. The second phase is resorption by osteoclasts which lasts about 15 days. The signal informing osteoclasts to stop digging the old matrix is not completely elucidated. Then comes the reversal phase: osteoblast precursors start to fill the resorption cavity. The growth factors stored in the bone matrix, are released in an active form during osteoclastic bone resorption and can subsequently stimulate osteoblast proliferation. They could therefore be involved in the physiological "coupling" between resorption and formation.

This "coupling" between resorption and formation is dependent on local factors released by osteoclasts from the ancient matrix. Indeed the last phase is apposition of new matrix by osteoblasts and complete filling of the cavity by new matrix. This process leads to maintenance of bone mass and an equilibrated balance between resorption and formation.

Cortical and Trabecular Bone

Diaphyses are made of cortical bone whereas metaphyses (extremities of the long bones and vertebral bodies) are made of trabecular bone. Cortical and trabecular bone remodeling are described in Table 1.1. The number of bone remodeling units per volume is 20 times higher in trabecular than in cortical bone due to the higher size of the remodeling units in cortical bone. By contrast, as the whole skeleton is made for 90% of cortical bone, the number of remodeling units in the trabecular bone is only 3 time higher than in the cortical bone. Vertebrae consist of 50% trabecular bone, and 50% cortical bone, and femoral neck consist of 30% trabecular and 70% cortical bone.

Table 1.1. Differences in bone remodeling in cortical and in trabecular bone (from M. Parfitt).

	Cortical bone	Trabecular bone
Number of bone remodeling units		
per mm^2 bone tissue	0.2	4
in the skeleton	0.3×10^5	1.4×10^5
Number of remodeling units		
activated each hour	100	760
Renewal (% per year)	3–4	25

The activation frequency is a lot higher in trabecular as compared to cortical bone due to the higher interface of trabecular bone with the marrow which is the origin of both type of bone cells. The integration of all these data, explain that the renewal of trabecular bone is 5 to 8 times higher in trabecular bone. Therefore the consequence of a desequilibrium in the bone balance will be apparent earlier in trabecular (vertebrae) than in cortical (femoral neck) bone.

2

Physiology of Calcium Homeostasis and Bone Remodeling

Dirk Vanderschueren & Roger Bouillon

Normal Calcium Homeostasis

Plasma ionized calcium (Ca^{++}) is regulated within narrow limits. Only 43% of total plasma calcium (normal concentration between 8.3 and 10.3 mg/dl) is ionized, another 10% is complexed to anions and the majority is bound to protein (90% to albumin). Normal concentrations of plasma ionized calcium therefore range between 1.8 and 3.0 mg/dl.

Calcium in plasma and extracellular fluid (the central pool of calcium) is less than 2% of total body calcium. The bulk of total body calcium (as for magnesium and phosphate) is present in the skeleton. The endoskeleton is composed of crystalline molecules such as hydroxyapatite $Ca_{10}(PO_4)_6(OH)_2$, which provides mechanical support and serves as a reservoir for the central pool of calcium.

This central pool of calcium has large fluxes across three epithelia (bone, kidney and intestine) which are regulated and modulated by the calciotropic hormones (Figure 2.1).

Adults in zero **net** calcium balance do not have **net** daily flux between the central calcium pool and bone. Thus urinary (plus sweat) calcium equals the daily net calcium absorption from intestine. Major deviations from zero calcium balance occur during skeletal growth, bone senescence, lactation and during disease.

The Calciotropic Hormones

Parathyroid Hormone (PTH)

PTH is the major hormone of calcium homeostasis. PTH is secreted by the parathyroid gland which serves as the central detector of plasma calcium by a specific membrane bound G-protein coupled calcium receptor.

The principal storage form in parathyroid secretory vesicles is the native hormone which consists of 84 amino acids. Although for full biological activity (binding to PTH-receptor), only the 34 amino terminal acids are needed, PTH circulates in its 1–84 form together with carboxy-terminal fragments that lack any relevant biological activity. Plasma calcium is the major modulator of PTH

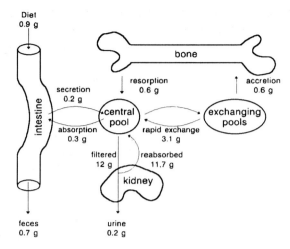

Figure 2.1. The central pool of calcium has large fluxes across the kidney, intestine and bone. The figure shows daily fluxes in balance for a diet of 900 mg.

secretion. When plasma calcium increases, PTH secretion is inhibited within seconds. PTH gene transcription and replication of parathyroid cell mass are also decreased by both calcium and $1,25(OH)_2D_3$, respectively in a scale of hours and weeks.

PTH acts to increase plasma Ca^{++} concentration in three ways:
- In the presence of permissive amounts of active Vitamin D, it stimulates bone resorption, resulting in release of calcium and phosphate.
- It enhances intestinal Ca^{++} and phosphate absorption indirectly by promoting the production of calcitriol in the kidney.
- It augments active renal Ca^{++} reabsorption in the distal tubule.

PTH also reduces proximal tubular reabsorption of phosphate. On the other hand, PTH tends to increase phosphate entry in the extracellular fluid by its effect on bone and intestinal absorption. However, the urinary effect of PTH on phosphate usually predominates. Therefore it mostly tends to lower serum phosphate.

Vitamin D

Vitamin D (cholecalciferol) results from conversion of 7-dehydrocholesterol in the skin, during exposure to solar ultraviolet irradiation. Cholecalciferol (vitamin D_3) must be distinguished from ergocalciferol (vitamin D_2) which is produced by ultraviolet irradiation of the fungal steroid ergosterol. Following the photochemical conversion of 7-dehydrocholesterol to vitamin D, it is transported in plasma bound to a vitamin D binding globulin. Before exerting biological effects, vitamin D undergoes a series of further metabolic conversions. The first step involves its hepatic conversion to a 25-hydroxylated derivative [$25(OH)D_3$], the major circulating metabolite and vitamin D store in the body. Subsequently, the renal 1α-hydroxylase enzyme converts $25(OH)D_3$ to the biologically active form $1,25(OH)_2D_3$ (1,25-dihydroxy-vitamin D or calcitriol).

The main regulators of $1,25(OH)_2D_3$ synthesis are the serum concentrations of $1,25(OH)_2D_3$ itself, calcium (calcemia), phosphate (phosphatemia) and PTH. PTH is the major inducer of the renal $25(OH)D_3$-1α-hydroxylase. Calcium is both a direct and an indirect regulator of this enzyme but its indirect effect through regulation of PTH is the more potent of the two.

The principal effects of $1,25(OH)_2D_3$ on calcium metabolism are to increase intestinal absorption of calcium and phosphate by inducing the synthesis of several proteins, including a specific calcium binding protein and a Ca-ATPase involved in intracellular calcium transport and serosal calcium uptake, respectively.

Vitamin D is also needed for appropriate bone mineralisation but, whether this is mainly an indirect effect via raising serum calcium and phosphorus or the result of direct stimulation of osteoblasts, is not firmly established. Bone resorption, however, is also stimulated by $1,25(OH)_2D_3$ especially since this hormone is the most powerful stimulus for osteoclast differentiation. Other target tissues are the parathyroid glands, where $1,25(OH)_2D_3$ suppresses the formation of PTH, and the kidney, where the main effect of $1,25(OH)_2D_3$ is downregulation of its own synthesis by suppression of 1α-hydroxylase as well as induction of 24-hydroxylase activity, which is the first step in the vitamin D catabolic pathway.

Calcitonin

Calcitonin is a 32-amino-acid polypeptide. Calcitonin is secreted by the parafollicular cells of the thyroid gland. The major stimulus of calcitonin is calcium. Calcitonin directly inhibits calcium and phosphate resorption by the osteoclasts. However, at physiological rates of bone resorption, the effects of calcitonin are only minimal. The major effects of the calciotropic hormones are summarized in Figure 2.2.

Bone Composition

Bone is made up essentially of mineral, organic matrix, cells and water. The mineral amounts to about two-thirds of the total dry weight of bone. It is made of small crystals which chemically contain mainly hydroxyapatite. The organic bone matrix amounts to about 35% of the dry weight of bone. It consists of 90% collagen, which provides bone its tensile strength by a complex three-dimensional structure, comparable to that of a rope. The remainder of the bone matrix is made of various non-collageneous proteins. The most abundant ones are osteonectin, osteocalcin, also called bone gla-protein (BGP), osteopontin and bone sialoprotein.

There are 4 major types of bone cells: osteoblasts, lining cells, osteocytes and osteoclasts. The **osteoblasts**, which derive from mesenchymal stem cells located in the bone marrow, are the cells that synthesize the osseous organ bone matrix. In a second step, this matrix calcifies extracellularly. Modulation of bone formation may occur at the level of the recruitment of new osteoblasts as well as through the alteration of osteoblast function, not only calciotropic and sex hormones *in vitro*, but also the insulin-like growth factors (IGFs), transforming growth factor (TGF-β), acidic and basic fibroblast growth factors (FGFs), platelet-derived growth factor (PDGF), bone morphogenetic proteins (BMPs) and prostaglandins, influence bone formation *in vitro*, but their role *in vivo* is not yet clear. In contrast, corticosteroids inhibit bone formation.

When the osteoblasts are not in the process of forming bone matrix, they are flat and therefore called resting osteoblasts or **lining cells**. Both active and resting osteoblasts form a membrane at the surface of the bone tissue.

Some osteoblasts are embedded within bone during the process of bone formation and mineralization. They are then called **osteocytes**. They are located in lacunae and interconnected by long cytoplasmic processes among themselves and with osteoblasts. Gap junctions at the membrane contact sites make a functional syncytium, allowing bone to respond to stimuli over large areas. These cell processes are located within canaliculi, which contain, together with the lacunae, the so-called bone fluid. As the surface of these lacunae and canaliculi is very large, in humans about 1000 m^2, the bone fluid is in immediate contact with the mineral, with which it is in equilibrium. The osteocytes are thought to influence the composition of this bone fluid and therefore may also play a role in calcium regulation. Osteocytes are also well located for responding to mechanical stress and may play a key role in translating mechanical stress into changes of bone formation and bone resorption.

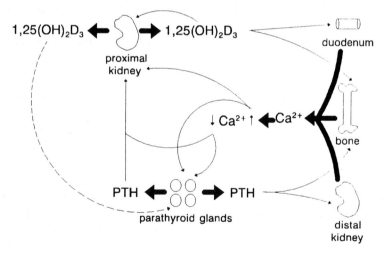

Figure 2.2. The major calciotropic hormones PTH and $1,25(OH)_2D_3$ constitute an integrated endocrine unit. It involves calcium sensing by the parathyroid gland, cooperative action of PTH and $1,25(OH)_2D_3$, modulation of calcium fluxes across duodenum, bone and distal kidney, feedback on PTH and $1,25(OH)_2D_3$ synthesis by calcium and $1,25(OH)_2D_3$.

The fourth type of cell in bone is the **osteoclast**. It originates from the hematopoietic compartment, more precisely from the granulocyte-macrophage colony-forming unit (GM-CFU). Osteoclasts are usually large multinucleated cells that are situated either on the surface or within the cortical or at the trabecular bone, often in depressions called Howship's lacunae. Within the cortical bone, osteoclasts are located at the tip of the remodeling units, burring the vascular canals in which the new osteons will be formed. Osteoclasts resorb bone in a sealed-off microenvironment located between the cell and the bone. Bone resorption can be modulated by altering either the recruitment of new osteoclasts or the activity of mature osteoclasts. Both processes seem to be under the control of the cells of osteoblastic lineage, which synthesize some factors such as cytokines, acting directly on the osteoclasts and/or their precursors.

The three main hormones modulating bone resorption are parathyroid hormone (PTH), $1,25$ $(OH)_2$ vitamin D_3 (calcitriol) and calcitonin, the first two increasing, the latter decreasing resorption. Furthermore, estrogens in women and testosterone in men inhibit bone resorption, in part at least by decreasing the production of interleukin (IL-6). Menopause and ovariectomy, as well as orchidectomy, induce a dramatic increase in bone resorption, probably mediated by an increase in IL-6.

Not only IL-6 but also the interleukins -1, -3 and -11 (IL-1, IL-3, IL-11), tumor necrosis factor-α and -β (TNF-α, TNF-β), macrophage colony-stimulating factor (M-CSF), granulocyte-macrophage colony-stimulating factor (GM-CSF), stem cell factor (SCF) and prostaglandins may increase bone resorption *in vitro*. Interferon-γ (IFN-γ), TGF-β, IL-4 and IL-13 on the other hand, decrease bone resorption. Some of these cytokines are produced by the cells of osteoblastic lineage and therefore possibly involved in the osteoblast-osteoclast interaction.

Modeling and Remodeling

Bone is continuously being turned over by the two processes of **modeling** and remodeling. In the former, new bone is formed at a location different from the one destroyed, resulting in a change in the shape of the skeleton during growth. It therefore allows not only the development of a normal architecture during growth, but also the adaptation of skeletal architecture to mechanical stress in the adult. Furthermore, it increases the size of the vertebrae during adult life. In **remodeling**, which is the main process in the adult, bone resorption and formation occur in the same place without change in the shape of bone. Both modeling and remodeling, however, result in the replacement of old by new bone. This allows both the maintenance of the mechanical integrity of the skeleton and assures its role as an ion bank.

The remodeling rate is between 2% and 10% of the skeletal mass per year. It is increased by parathyroid hormone, thyroxine, growth hormone and $1,25(OH)_2$ vitamin D_3, decreased by calcitonin, estrogen and glucocorticosteroids. It is also stimulated by microfractures and mechanical stress. The cancellous bone, which represents about 20% of the skeletal mass, makes up 80% of the turnover, while

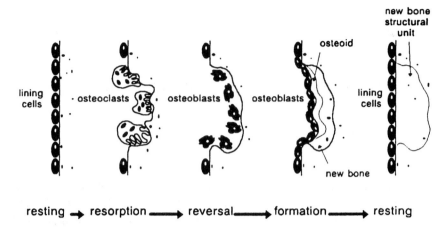

resting → resorption ———→ reversal ———→ formation ———→ resting

Figure 2.3. Bone remodelling occurs in different phases. During the resorption osteoclasts replace the lining cells. During the reversal phase, osteoblasts replace osteoclasts and form osteoid that is mineralized thereafter. Finally, a new bone structural unit is formed.

the cortex, which represents 80% of the bone, makes up only 20% of the turnover. The morphological dynamic substrate of bone turnover is the "bone multicellular unit" (BMU) or "bone remodeling unit" (BRU). The morphological entity formed when the process is terminated is called the "bone structural unit" (BSU) which corresponds to the packet in cancellous bone, and to the osteon in cortical bone. Both in the cortex and in the trabeculae, the first step of bone remodeling is activation of osteoclasts which erode bone. In a second step, the resorption sites are refilled by the osteoblasts.

Normally, the amount of bone formed equals the amount destroyed, so that the balance is zero. The bone remodeling process is illustrated in Figure 2.3.

Summary

- Calcium homeostasis is dependent on 3 major organs (intestine, kidney and bone) and on 3 major hormones (PTH, $1,25(OH)_2D_3$, and calcitonin).
- Bone composition is complex and contains matrix with minerals and proteins (collagen and others)
- Bone is continuously turned over by osteoclasts and osteoblasts, during growth by modeling and during adulthood by remodeling.

3

Biomechanics of Bone and Fracture

Lis Mosekilde

The incidence of vertebral fractures has increased three- to fourfold for women and more than fourfold for men during the last 30 years. In the UK and Scandinavia, fractures of the femoral neck have shown the same pattern, with a two- to threefold increase in incidence for both men and women. The data are age-adjusted and therefore highlight the decrease in bone mass or bone quality from generation to generation. To arrest or reverse these increases in osteoporotic fractures, effective preventive regimens must be established. However, in order to do so, a basic understanding of age-related changes in the quality and strength of vertebral bone and of the femoral neck is crucial.

Vertebrae

Normal Age-related Changes

When peak bone mass has been attained, at the age of 25–30 years, the vertebral body consists of a central trabecular network demarcated by a bony shell of approximately 400–500 μm thick. The cortical thickness and the density of the trabecular network are identical for young men and women, but the cross-sectional area is 25–30% larger in men. This difference in cross-sectional area leads to a higher bone mass in men and also to a higher strength (or loadbearing capacity). In young individuals, the loading capacity of a lumbar vertebral body is of the order of 1,000 kg, or even more in men (Figure 3.1a).

With age, the density and architecture of the internal trabecular bone change as a result of the remodeling process (which has a slightly negative balance). Concomitantly, there is a thinning of both the endplates and the cortical shell due to endosteal resorption of bone. As a result of these changes, the loadbearing capacity of the vertebral body is reduced to only 120–150 kg in an elderly individual. The decline in cortical thickness and in trabecular density are identical for men and women, but during normal aging there is a male-specific increase in cross-sectional area of the vertebral bodies. The modeling process causes this increase in cross-sectional area through periosteal apposition, and it acts as a compensatory mechanism for the age-related decline in bone density (Figure 3.1b).

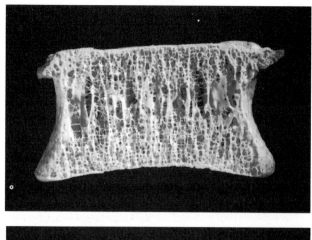

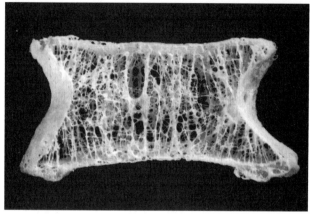

Figure 3.1. (a) The vertebral body of a young individual. The trabecular network is dense and well-connected. (b) The vertebral body of an elderly individual. There is a loss of density and of structural integrity

Osteoporosis

In osteoporosis, the normal age-related changes in cortical thickness and trabecular bone density and connectivity become even more pronounced. The sum of these changes causes an extreme weakening of the vertebral bodies. The loadbearing capacity of whole lumbar vertebrae often declines to values around 60–90 kg (i.e. a reduction from "peak" of around 90%). In osteoporotic patients, the cortical thickness declines to values around 120–150 μm. The central trabecular architecture changes with loss of connectivity, due to osteoclastic perforations of the thin horizontal trabeculae (Figure 3.2a), and with formation of microcalluses on vertical trabecular structures due to overloading and microfractures (Figure 3.2b).

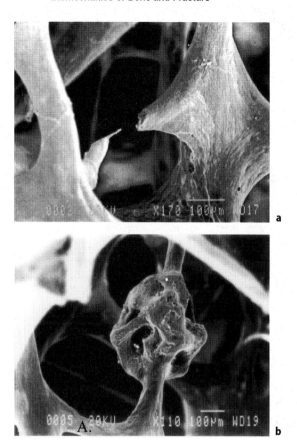

Figure 3.2. (a) Scanning electron microscopy showing osteoclastic perforation of a horizontal strut (the footprints of the osteoclast are still visible). (b) Scanning electron microscopy of a microcallus (early healing microfracture) located typically on a vertical trabecula.

The radiographic picture of such changes shows, primarily, an extremely thin structure of the vertebral trabecular network, with a predominance of vertical structures. Thereafter, small endplate depressions appear, as a result of thin endplates and the weakened trabecular structure beneath. The next stage is, typically, biconcave vertebrae followed first by wedge shaped vertebral bodies and finally by complete compression fractures.

The strength of vertebral bone in osteoporotic patients is determined by both trabecular and cortical bone, but because the trabecular network has almost totally disappeared at this stage, the cortical ring assumes relatively more importance (Table 3.1). As in normal individuals, the size of the vertebral body is important for its loadbearing capacity, and several studies have shown that osteoporotic women typically have small vertebral bodies.

Table 3.1. Characteristic age-related changes in vertebral trabecular bone density, cortical thickness, strength, and strength of the cortex as a percentage of total strength.

Age (years)	20–40	70–80	Osteoporotic
Density (g/cm^3)	0.200–0.250	0.100–0.150	0.060–0.090
Cortical thickness (mm)	400–500	200–300	120–150
Strength (kg)	1000–1200	150–250	60–150
Strength of cortical rim (% of total)	25–30	70–80	80–90

The ratio between vertebral fractures in men and women was previously thought to be 1: 10, but new data show that this is incorrect and that the ratio is near 1: 2.

The reason for this sex-specific difference can be explained by the differences in the aging pattern of men and women: (1) men achieve a higher peak bone mass than in women, mainly because of the larger cross-sectional area of their bones (25–30% larger than in women); (2) men have no accelerated bone loss in middle age; (3) men seem to be able to compensate for loss of bone material strength by increasing vertebral cross-sectional area with age; in addition, (4) men seem to have less tendency to trabecular perforation than women.

Femoral Neck

Normal Age-related Changes

Like the vertebral bodies, the femoral neck consists of a central trabecular network and a relatively thin cortical shell.

The age-related changes at the femoral neck site are identical to those described at the vertebral body site: a decline in trabecular density and connectivity and a thinning of the cortical shell.

The femoral neck is very special, however, in that part of the neck is placed intracapsularly – this means that it is not covered by periosteal tissue – and therefore it cannot increase in size during normal aging due to periosteal apposition. For this reason, loading of the femoral neck might not prevent cervical fractures (intracapsularly) but only affect intertrochanteric fractures (extracapsularly).

Fractures

The femoral neck fracture also differs from the vertebral fracture by always being related to a trauma (e.g. a fall). Therefore, fracture incidence at this site is related not only to bone strength as such, but also to muscle strength and balance. The ratio between femoral neck fracture in men and women is 1: 2.5, but some of this ratio might well be explained by the fact that women fall twice as often as men.

The Importance of Loading for Maintenance of Bone Mass, Structure and Strength

Loading affects the human skeleton through two different mechanisms: remodeling and modeling.

The remodeling process, which causes thinning and perforation of the trabecular structures, will increase dramatically during immobilization (leading to bone loss of 60–70% within 6 months). However, loading the skeleton against gravity a few times daily will delay the remodeling process and thereby reduce the extreme loss of bone mass.

Vigorous, daily exercise or sport might even be able to arrest the normal age-related bone loss by decreasing activation of the remodeling process.

The modeling process adds new bone to the periosteal surfaces; loading stimulates the process, leading to bones with larger cross-sectional areas and thicker cortices. Loading of the skeleton thereby leads to stronger bones and a decline in fracture liability.

Summary

Strength of vertebral bone and of the femoral neck is determined by several factors, including cortical thickness, trabecular bone density, architecture, and bone size. All these factors change with age as a result of the remodeling process.

When the changes become pronounced, osteoporotic fractures occur. Although there are differences in the aging patterns between men and women, the general pattern for both sexes is identical and leads to an extreme loss of bone strength (70–80%). In osteoporosis, this loss of bone strength might well amount to 90% of "peak bone strength".

Loading plays an important role in the maintenance of trabecular connectivity (through the remodeling process) and in the periosteal apposition (through the modeling process). Loading is therefore important for the maintenance of bone strength during normal aging – and exercise plays an important role in the prevention of osteoporotic fractures.

4

Epidemiology of Osteoporosis

Richard W. Keen & Tim D. Spector

Osteoporosis is a common skeletal disease characterized by low bone mass, deterioration of skeletal architecture and an increased susceptibility to fragility fracture. Osteoporotic fractures tend to occur at skeletal sites with a high trabecular bone content, with common fractures being in the thoracic and lumbar spines, the hip and at the wrist. These fractures are characterized by higher incidence rates in women compared to men, and a sharp rise in the fracture rates with increasing age. The lifetime risk for these common osteoporotic fractures in British men and women is shown in Table 4.1. Fracture incidence in the community shows a bimodal distribution with age, with peaks in youth and the elderly. Fractures in the young commonly affect long bones due to major trauma and their incidence is consequently higher in males compared to females.

Table 4.1. Lifetime risk of the common osteoporotic-related fractures in U.K. men and women aged 50 years.

	Men (%)	Women (%)
Hip	3	14
Vertebral (spine) *	2	11
Distal forearm (wrist)	2	13

*Data for clinically diagnosed vertebral deformity.

Low bone mineral density (BMD) is implicit in the definition of osteoporosis, and is a strong predictor for subsequent fracture. The World Health Organization has devised definitions for established osteoporosis (BMD 2.5 standard deviations below the peak, young normal mean), and with these definitions it has been possible to estimate the prevalence of osteoporosis within populations. In the U.K. the prevalence of established osteoporosis in women aged 50–54 years is 3.5% at the lumbar spine and 2.0% at the femoral neck. These prevalence rates are age-dependent, such that at the age of 70–74 years these figures have risen to 15% at the spine and 20% at the hip.

Hip Fracture

Hip fractures represent the most serious of osteoporotic fractures, with an excess mortality at 6 months and a major associated morbidity in survivors. The average age when a hip fracture occurs in the UK is 79 years with most of these occurring after a fall from a standing height or less. Potential modifiable factors in the etiology of hip fracture include the frequency of falls, the individual's response to the fall, and impaired skeletal structure and strength. There is a world-wide seasonal variation in hip fracture, with the highest occurrence being in the winter. This may be a consequence of the icy conditions increasing the likelihood of falls, a cold induced reduction in neuromuscular response to falls or to reduced vitamin D levels due to low sunlight exposure. Hip fractures are commonest in Northern European countries and from their descendents in North America. Most countries have seen a doubling in rates of hip fracture over the last 30 years although rates now appear to be plateauing.

Vertebral Fracture

Vertebral fractures are commonly asymptomatic and prevalence estimates can only be reliably obtained by radiological survey of the thoracolumbar spine although there remains a lack of a universally accepted definition for vertebral deformity and fracture. Recent data from the European Vertebral Osteoporosis Study has suggested an overall prevalence of vertebral deformity of approximately 12% in both sexes. Spinal deformity was more common in younger males compared to females, probably as a consequence of occupation and trauma. This difference in prevalence rates between the sexes was reversed in old age, with women showing a steeper gradient in this age-related increase. Vertebral deformities are also associated with reduced life expectancy, probably as a consequence of pre-existing comorbid conditions.

Forearm Fracture

Forearm fracture incidence rates in women increase linearly from age 40–65 years and then plateau, whereas in males the incidence remains constant between 20 and 80 years. The age-adjusted sex ratio for these fractures is 4: 1 (female to male), which is more marked than for both hip and vertebral fractures. There is a seasonal variation in the incidence of wrist fractures, which is more clearly associated with falls onto an out-stretched arm during the winter months.

Risk Factors

Risk factors for osteoporosis and fracture include factors influencing bone mass, skeletal architecture, and tendency for falls. Many studies have identified epidemiological risk factors that are associated with these at the population level, although these risk factors appear too insensitive to act as predictive or diagnostic tools for individual subjects (Table 4.2). It remains to be determined however whether any of these risk factors can be modified in a cost-effective manner to significantly reduce the incidence of osteoporosis and the healthcare burden of fracture.

Table 4.2. Epidemiological risk factors for
osteoporosis and fracture.

Age
Premature menopause
History of amenorrhea
Low body mass index
History of anorexia nervosa
History of hyperthyroidism
Smoking
Alcohol intake
Caffeine intake
Current use of benzodiazepines
Current use of anti-convulsants
Low exercise levels
Inability to rise from chair
Previous fractures
History of maternal hip fracture
Low bone density
Increased hip axis length
Low quantitative ultrasound measurement

Family and twin studies have demonstrated a strong genetic component to osteoporosis, with 60–85% of the population variation in BMD being attributable to genetic factors. Maternal history of hip fracture is associated with a 2-fold increased risk of hip fracture, and similar increases in the risk of wrist fracture are seen in those with a positive history of fracture at this in first-degree relatives. The genetic influence on osteoporosis risk may also have an influence on other known risk factors such as skeletal size, hip geometry, bone architecture and muscle strength.

Conclusion

Over the next 50 years the number of hip fractures in all countries will continue to increase due to an aging population. Osteoporosis is a complex multifactorial disease which remains asymptomatic until a fracture occurs and strategies need to be developed to accurately identify "high risk" subjects who may benefit from preventive treatments before the fracture occurs. Strategies for this may include combinations of risk factor profiles, bone density or bone structure measurements, bone markers or genetic markers. Understanding the epidemiology of osteoporosis and fracture risk may therefore ultimately aid in reducing the public health burden of this common disease.

Summary

Osteoporosis is a complex disease characterized by reduced bone mass, deterioration in skeletal architecture and an increased fracture risk. Common osteoporotic fractures occur at the hip, thoracolumbar spine and wrist (Colles' fracture).

The incidence of osteoporotic fractures increases with age in both sexes. For white Caucasian women the lifetime risk for experiencing any osteoporotic-related fracture is 30%. The lifetime risk in males is approximately 1/4 that of females.

Fracture incidence is highest in those of Northern European background with lower rates being observed in other racial groups such as Afro-Carribeans. Fracture rates can however vary within countries with populations of the same racial background, suggesting the action of unique environmental factors.

Hip fractures will increase in all countries over the next 30–50 years due to both an aging population and to an increase in the age-adjusted hip fracture incidence.

The risk factor profiles for the 3 main osteoporotic fractures show both common epidemiological risk factors and also factors that appear site specific. Knowledge of these factors may accurately identify "high risk" subjects.

Modification of key epidemiological risk factors may lead to a reduction in osteoporotic fracture and will ultimately reduce the burden of this common disease.

Suggested Reading

Arden NK, Baker J, Hogg C, Baan K, Spector TD. (1996) The heritability of bone mineral density, ultrasound of the calcaneus and hip axis length: a study of postmenopausal twins. *J Bone Min Res* 11: 530–534.

Consensus Development Conference. (1993) Diagnosis, prophylaxis and treatment of osteoporosis. *Am J Med* 94: 646–650.

Compston JE, Cooper C, Kanis JA. (1995) Bone densitometry in clinical practice. *BMJ* 310: 1507–1510.

Cummings SR, Nevitt MC, Browner WS et al. (1995) Risk factors for hip fracture in white women. *N Engl J Med* 332: 767–773.

Hans D, Dargent-Molina P, Schott AM et al. (1996) Ultrasonographic heel measurements to predict hip fracture in elderly women: the EPIDOS prospective study. *Lancet* 348: 511–514.

Mallmin H, Ljunghall S, Persson I, Bergstrom R. (1994) Risk factors for fractures of the distal forearm: a population-based case-control study. *Osteoporosis Int* 4: 298–304.

Nguyen T, Sambrook P, Kelly P et al. (1993) Prediction of osteoporotic fractures by potural instability and bone density. *BMJ* 307: 1111–1115.

O'Neil TW, Felsenberg D, Varlow et al. (1996) The prevalence of vertebral deformity in European men and women: the European Vertebral Osteoporosis Study. *J Bone Miner Res* 11: 1010–1018.

Reid IR, Chin KC, Evans MC, Jones JG. (1994) Relation between increase in length of hip axis in older women between 1950s and 1990s and increase in age specific rates of hip fracture. *BMJ* 309: 508–509.

Seeman E, Hopper JL, Bach, LA, Cooper ME, Parkinson E, McKay J, Jerums G. (1989) Reduced bone mass in daughters of women with osteoporosis. *N Engl J Med* 320: 554–558.

Spector TD, Edwards AC, Thompson PW. (1992) Use of a risk factor and dietary calcium questionnaire in predicting bone density and subsequent bone loss at the menopause. *Ann Rheum Dis* 51: 1252–1253.

5

Pathophysiology of Fractures

Michael R. McClung

Fractures are the complication of osteoporosis much as strokes are the complication and result of hypertension. It is only through fractures that osteoporosis manifests its clinical effects or has clinical relevance. Fractures occur in patients with decreased bone strength who experience an injury. Thus the pathophysiology of fractures encompasses a multitude of factors which determine bone strength (bone mass, bone quality, age and skeletal geometry) and the frequency, nature of and effects of injuries (Figure 5.1). Each of these factors becomes more prevalent with advancing age, resulting in the exponential increase in the prevalence of fractures related to osteoporosis in elderly individuals. Understanding the determinants of fracture risk provides the basis of appropriate and effective interventions to reduce fracture frequency and the complications of osteoporosis.

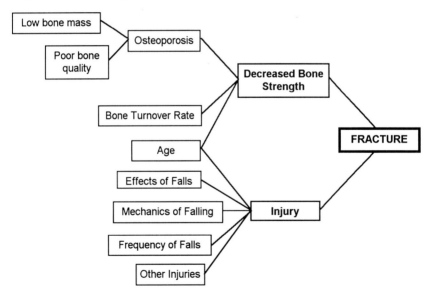

Figure 5.1. Determinants of fracture risk. Both skeletal and non-skeletal factors are important predictors and determinants of fracture risk.

Peak Bone Mass

The level of bone mass in adults is determined by the level of peak bone mass acquired during skeletal maturation and by the rate and duration of bone loss which occurs thereafter. Peak bone mass is attained by age 20–25 and is influenced by both genetic and environmental factors. The role of hereditary in determining peak bone mass is dominant and accounts for 60–80% of the variance in peak bone mass. The effect is in part related to body size and build, but is also related to other factors. Peak bone mass can be optimized by various environmental factors including nutrition (especially calcium and caloric intake), physical activity, and sex steroid status. The combined effects of heredity and these environmental factors can be modified by medical problems such as anticonvulsant and glucocorticoid use, intestinal malabsorption, type I diabetes, and chronic inflammatory conditions.

Increased calcium intake in children and adolescents results in a modest increase in bone mass, but the extent to which this effects final peak bone mass is not yet clear. Growing children and young adults who habitually are more physically active have higher bone mass than their sedentary peers. Young adults of both genders who experience a delay in puberty or transient intervals of sex steroid deficiency after puberty seem to have lower peak bone mass.

Bone Loss

Following the acquisition of skeletal maturity, bone mass is relatively stable during young adult years, although some longitudinal studies suggests a very slow rate of bone loss beginning as early as age 30 in both men and women. The determinants of bone loss in healthy premenopausal women and young men, if it occurs, are not known. In women, a clear change in skeletal status occurs at menopause. As a consequence of estrogen deficiency, the rate of bone turnover increases and the imbalance between resorption and formation widens. As a result, bone loss accelerates to about 2% per year (measured by absorptiometric techniques). Within about five years, the rate of bone loss gradually slows to <1% per year. Recent studies demonstrate that the rate of bone loss again accelerates in advanced age, perhaps as a result of acquired inefficiencies of calcium balance including decreased intake of calcium and vitamin D, decreased solar exposure, impaired renal activation of vitamin D, and intestinal resistance to active vitamin D metabolites. Indeed, older individuals frequently have subclinical vitamin D deficiency and/or secondary hyperparathyroidism which may drive osteoclastic bone resorption and bone loss. This may explain the observation that calcium and vitamin D administration seems to have greater effects on bone mineral density (BMD) in older women compared to those in early menopause.

Bone Mass and Fracture Risk

The relationship between bone mass and fracture risk has been well studied in women over age 65. As bone mass decreases, fracture risk increases exponentially (Figure 5.2a). For every standard deviation (SD) decrease in bone

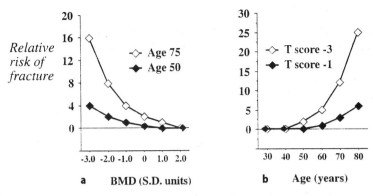

Figure 5.2. (a) The relationship between BMD and fracture risk is exponential and varies by the age of the individual. (b) Fracture risk increases with age even if BMD remains stable.

density, the risk of osteoporotic fracture increases by a factor of 1.5–2. The risk of hip fracture is even more strongly predicted by measuring bone density in the proximal femur, for hip fracture risk increases by 2.6 fold for every SD decrease in hip density. The relationship between bone mass and fracture risk is at least as strong as the relationship between blood pressure elevation and the risk of stroke and is much stronger than the association of serum cholesterol levels and the risk of heart attack.

The nature of the relationship between bone density and fracture risk is such that a relatively large decrease in BMD from young normal values is required before fracture risk becomes clinically significant. However, in patients with very low bone mass, quite small changes result in significant changes in fracture risk. This in part may explain the large reduction in fracture incidence afforded by pharmacologic treatments which cause only small changes in bone density in patients with osteoporosis.

Since the relationship between bone density and fracture risk is exponential, there is no true "fracture threshold", a level of bone density where fractures begin to occur. Rather, there is a progressive increase in fracture risk as bone density declines. From a clinical perspective, however, fractures related to osteoporosis are uncommon in individuals whose bone density is within 2.5 SD of the average young adult values, while individuals with BMD values below this value are at quite high risk of experiencing a fracture over the next few years. This then is the basis of the definitions of osteoporosis (such as that of the World Health organization) based solely on BMD values.

Bone Quality

As bone loss occurs, architectural changes accrue that further impair skeletal strength. The number of trabecular plates decreases as does the "connectedness" of the trabecular network. The relative importance of bone mass versus bone "quality" is difficult to determine, since practical methods of assessing bone quality are not available. By the time clinical osteoporosis is evident, bone quality is impaired. How much bone mass must decrease before these architectural changes begin to occur is not known. The answer to this question will have potential importance in determining the most appropriate and optimal time to intervene with agents to prevent progression of bone loss and the deterioration of bone quality. In addition to the macroscopic architectural changes, more subtle changes in bone quality may occur due to the accumulation of microdamage within the bone. As this structural damage occurs, bone fragility increases. The normal bone remodeling process minimizes this problem by repairing this microdamage. In patients with low turnover forms of osteoporosis, the accumulation of microdamage may be a very important component of skeletal fragility.

Bone Remodeling

In addition to its effect on BMD, an increased rate of bone remodeling appears to be a factor in fracture risk. Several studies now demonstrate that elevation of biochemical tests which reflect bone turnover or modulation of calcium metabolism are predictive of hip fractures in older women. These tests include biochemical markers of bone resorption (Type I collagen crosslinks) and bone formation (bone-specific alkaline phosphatase, osteocalcin), elevated parathyroid hormone and low serum 25(OH) vitamin D_3 levels. These tests not only demonstrate the pathogenesis of fracture risk but may be useful clinically in assessing the need of individual patients for therapeutic intervention and for monitoring the response to therapy.

Age

Age itself is an important predictor of fracture risk. The risk of fracture due to osteoporosis doubles every 5–7 years. Only part of this effect is related to bone density changes with age. Older individuals are at greater risk of fracture than are younger subjects with the same bone density (Figure 5.2b). The effects of aging on fracture risk are a combination of age-related changes in bone density and quality, bone turnover rate and the risk of injury. Whether there is a unique effect of aging in fracture risk other than these effects is unknown.

Skeletal Geometry

It is clear that bone mass is not the only skeletal factor which affects bone strength or fracture risk. The geometry of material properties is of substantial importance in determining strength (see Chapter 3). One easily measured geometric variable is the hip axis length described by Faulkner et al., a measure through the long axis of the femoral neck from the trochanter to the inner margin of the pelvis. This value can be obtained from the image of the standard DXA BMD test of the proximal femur. The measurement is predictive of hip fracture, independent of bone density and body size, and seems to be the most valuable of many measurements assessed in the proximal femur. Differences in hip geometry may explain, at least in part, the observation that Asian women experience fewer hip fractures than do Caucasian women, despite having lower bone mineral density, for the hip axis length is shorter in Asian compared to Caucasian women.

Previous Fractures

One of the strongest predictors of fracture risk is the presence of a previous osteoporotic fracture. Prevalent spine fractures increase the risk of subsequent fracture by two- to five-fold. Likewise, having one hip fracture is a risk factor for subsequent fractures of the other hip, and having a wrist or spine fracture also increases the risk of subsequent hip fracture. The mechanism of this effect is not known. It is independent of BMD, but may reflect altered bone quality or the presence of other extraskeletal risk factors. At least in the spine, the alteration of skeletal mechanics and loading characteristics of vertebrae adjacent to the fracture site is a likely component of this effect. A maternal history of hip fracture is also an independent risk factor for hip fracture in older women.

Injury

While patients with osteoporosis are at risk for increased fracture, not all patients with osteoporosis experience fracture. Almost all fractures due to osteoporosis occur after an injury, albeit minor. Most hip fractures (>90%) occur as a result of a fall (very few hip fractures occur spontaneously, causing the fall). About 50% of spine fractures are also related to falls. Fall frequency increases with aging. Many studies have identified clinical risk factors predictive of falls (Table 5.1) or fractures (Table 5.2).

Table 5.1. Important risk factors for falls.

Use of sedatives
Cognitive impairment
Lower extremity disability
Palmomental reflex
Foot problems
Disturbances of gait and balance

Many of the determinants and predictors of falls are also known to be risk factors for fracture, underscoring the importance of falls in the pathogenesis of osteoporotic fractures. Incorporating an assessment of these risk factors for falls and fractures into daily clinical practice has two important roles. First, some of these risk factors for falls are correctable or modifiable, providing targets for therapeutic intervention with which to decrease fracture risk. Additionally, physicians can combine clinical risk factors with other measures such as BMD to more clearly stratify patients into gradations of risk. In one large study of hip fractures in elderly women, the great majority of hip fractures occurred in a small set of subjects who had multiple clinical risk factors for fracture <u>and</u> the lowest BMD.

Table 5.2. Important risk factors for fractures.

Thinness, loss of weight
Weakness
Smoking
Sedative medications
Neurologic diseases
Visual impairment
History of falling
Maternal hip fracture
Prior fragility fracture
Low bone mass

Types of Falls

The type of fall determines both the likelihood and the type of fracture. Falling forward usually results in a fracture of the distal radius. A fall into a sitting position may result in spinal fractures, while hip fractures most often occur when elderly subjects fall to the side, resulting in a strike to the trochanter. Individuals most likely to fall to the side are those who are frail and weak, have impaired balance, and who walk slowly. Recognition of such patients allows for appropriate interventions to decrease the frequency or effects of these fractures.

Fortunately, most falls do not result in a fracture. The ability of persons to protect themselves from the effects of a fall influence fracture risk. Individuals who are strong and who have better reflexes are less likely to sustain a fracture when they fall.

Other Injuries

Fractures of the spine and ribs often occur with other minor forms of trauma such as an injury while twisting or lifting or being hugged vigorously. Education about proper safety precautions and body mechanics is important to minimize these injuries.

Summary

There are multiple determinants of fractures, many of which are related to each other by virtue of there increased prevalence with aging. Osteoporosis (or low bone mass) is a major risk factor for fractures, but it is not the only factor. Appropriate strategies for decreasing fracture frequency will include both pharmacologic and nonpharmacologic approaches which address the wide variety of risk factors for fracture with which our patients present.

Suggested Reading

Cooper C et al. (1992) Incidence of clinically diagnosed vertebral fractures: a population-based study in Rochester, Minnesota, 1985–1989. *J Bone Miner Res* 7: 221–227.

Cummings SR et al. (1995) Risk factors for hip fracture in white women. *N Eng J Med* 332: 767–773.

Greenspan SL et al. (1994) Fall severity and bone mineral density as risk factors for hip fracture in ambulatory elderly. *JAMA* 271: 128–133.

Hui SL et al. (1988) Age and bone mass as predictors of fracture in a prospective study. *J Clin Invest* 81: 1804–1809.

Tinetti ME et al. (1988) Risk factors for falls among elderly persons living in the community. *N Eng J Med* 319: 1701–1707.

6

Short- and Long-term Outco
Osteoporotic Fractures

Anthony R. Lyons

Fractures taken as a whole increase in incidence with advancing age but those of the ankle, proximal forearm bones and digits have been shown to occur independently of the fall in bone mass associated with osteoporosis.

The most common fractures in osteoporotic patients are those of the distal radius (Colles' fracture), vertebral body and proximal femur. These will be considered in this chapter.

General Comments

Fractures in osteoporotic patients heal normally with formation of appropriate fracture callus and remodeled bone. Satisfactory internal fixation to allow early mobilization or weight bearing is sometimes difficult to achieve and this limits the application of the principles of osteosynthesis in these patients. Low demand elderly patients tolerate a greater degree of malunion than would be acceptable for a younger individual. Treatment aims to restore function (and therefore mobility) as soon as practicable to avoid the higher degree of morbidity and mortality seen in such patients with pre-existing co-morbidities. It should therefore be carried out by an experienced surgical and nursing team with expertise in dealing with osteoporotic patients.

Assessment of rehabilitation potential is vital for each individual case. Non-surgical therapy including physiotherapy and occupational therapy are prescribed as appropriate and are directed at achieving a satisfactory functional outcome. Currently available drug treatments for osteoporosis including hormone replacement therapy, bisphosphonates and calcium and vitamin D do not appear to adversely affect fracture healing if taken in the recommended manner and doses.

Vertebral Fractures

These fractures may occur spontaneously or as a result of minimal trauma. The most usual sites for fractures to occur is the thoraco-lumbar region (T11 – L4) and the mid-thoracic region (T5 – T8). The incidence is probably underestimated as many are asymptomatic. The proportion of all such fractures causing non-

pain is therefore unknown. Multiple fractures are associated with a
gree of morbidity than single fractures.

Short-term Outcome

Many fractures remain asymptomatic and are found only incidentally on X-rays
taken for investigation of chronic low back pain. Whilst fractures may indeed
cause pain, back pain per se is so common in those past retirement age it may be
attributable to other pathology.

Onset of well localized pain after varying degrees of trauma (with the pain felt
at the level of the fracture) occurring suddenly or over a very short (few days at
most) timespan is characteristic of an acute vertebral fracture. The site of the
vertebra affected and the radicular nature of the pain may differentiate it from
that of an acute disc protrusion. There is usually no bone tenderness to be felt on
palpation. The neurological signs are seldom sustained in the long term and only
very rarely lead to surgical intervention.

Fractured bone is a source of haemorrhage and this may be significant
(particularly in multiple fractures). This may affect the retroperitoneal space
leading to bowel ileus and abdominal distension.

During this period the patient may be disabled by the combination of pain and
paravertebral muscle spasm.

Medium-term Outcome

The acute pain and in particular associated radicular dermatomal pain may last
for several months. It may give way to chronic back ache as the biomechanics of
the back are altered by the new anatomical arrangements.

Long-term Morbidity

Repeated fractures lead to a loss of height and if of the wedge type seen
commonly in the dorsal spine may lead to the development of a kyphosis. This
increases the incidence of pulmonary complications by restricting thoracic
expansion, decreasing vital capacity and exercise tolerance.

The loss of abdominal cavity vertical height causes abdominal protrusion which
increases the likelihood of symptomatic hiatus hernia and other more non-
specific gastrointestinal symptoms. A kyphosis may lead to increased neck pain
and paravertebral muscle fatigue particularly if there is pre-existing degenerate
cervical spine disease.

Chronic pain and loss of normal body habitus may combine to cause
depression.

Mortality

Mortality increases after vertebral fracture although interpreting data is difficult
because of the associated co-morbidities. The increase is not seen immediately

after the fracture (and as discussed an unknown percentage of fractures are asymptomatic) but is continuous.

Hip fractures

The fractures usually occur as a result of mild trauma such as a simple fall. Almost all require surgical intervention as non-operative treatment is associated with the complications of immobilization including decubitus ulcers and pulmonary complications.

Mortality and morbidity are associated with the fall, hospitalization and co-morbidities.

Short-Term Outcome

Many patients are unable to summon help after falling and may be found hypothermic with a developing orthostatic pneumonia and decubitus ulcers all of which increase short term mortality. Hospital complications are common (>30%) and relate not only to the implants used in surgery (dislocation, fixation failure, infection) but also the complications of anaesthetic stress. They are correlated strongly with pre-surgery anaesthetic gradings (American Society of Anesthesiologists ASA Score). In-hospital mortality averages 10%.

Long-Term Outcome

Long term morbidity is high. A serious post-operative complication increases the 1 year mortality by a multiple of three. Functional recovery results remain poor as assessed with relation to mobility and dependency. Prospective case controlled data are scarce and suggest that between 41 and 97% of all fractures regain pre-fracture walking ability and this is positively associated with male sex, young age, absence of dementia or post-operative confusional state and somewhat counterintuitavely use of a walking aid prior to fracture. Implant specific complications including infection have been shown to reduce mobility but there is no clear relationship between type of fracture or type of implant 1 year after surgery.

Hip fracture patients constitute one of the groups of long stayers in any hospital system and the ability to return home is an increasingly important outcome measure. It is especially important when the reported data suggest that those who return home have a 40-fold chance of remaining alive at 10 years as compared to those institutionalized. Those at home sustain only a 31% reduction in social function as compared to a 55% reduction in those transferred to a rehabilitation center. Return to independence is predicted by age less than 85 years, pre-operatively being able to perform some activities of daily living, living with another and being able to walk independently at discharge.

Patients with no residual pain do better after a hip fracture. Intracapsular fractures are associated with less pain than extracapsular fractures and also do better if the femoral head is replaced rather than screwed *in situ* – a finding attributable to the stability of the implant in the femoral canal. It has been reported that at an average of 3.5 years follow up 45% of patients were still experiencing significant pain.

Mortality

Hip fracture is one clinical sign of declining general health. The death rates in patients sustaining a hip fracture exceed those of the general population. The death numbers are probably underreported but may be gleaned from follow up data of specific prostheses with an average of 30% one year mortality.

If case controlled studies are examined the overall true (over that expected) mortality approximates to 15%. The mortality rate has been constantly shown to be associated with poorly controlled systemic disease (especially four or more co-morbidities), cognitive dysfunction and operative intervention before stabilization of three or more co-morbidities. The associations between male sex, advanced age, institutionalization, fracture and anaesthetic type are less clear when co-morbidities are taken into consideration.

Fractures of the Distal Radius

In 1841 Benjamin Colles described his eponymous fracture of the distal radius but data from prospective studies relating function to treatment are scarce. Nevertheless these fractures are common, painful and may require operative intervention to place the bony fragments in the most anatomical position.

Assessment of outcome from published studies is difficult because of the differing classification systems used by authors. Reported results vary widely and are described here.

Functional Outcome

An analysis of over 1600 cases using the grading scale of Lindstrom showed that 76% of cases achieved a satisfactory result within 6 months of injury. However, many patients continue to complain of subjective symptoms – as many as 46% – 97% in one series.

Symptoms complained of include a feeling of weakness of the hand (2.3% – 6.6%), poor grip (18% – 35%) and persistent pain at the fracture site (24% – 75%).

Increasing age appears to lead to poorer functional results and younger patients (less than 64 yr.) have been demonstrated to regain movement more quickly. The original degree of dorsal tilt of the distal fragment (i.e. the initial displacement) or fracture pattern has been shown to have no effect upon the end result except results are inferior in severely comminuted intra-articular fractures. Even perfect anatomical reductions have been associated with a 2–5% poor functional result.

The residual dorsal tilt however has been shown to correlate with functional loss and the value of greater than 10^0 has been shown to lead to a greater than

40% unsatisfactory results. Angulation also significantly increases the loss of grip strength.

Complications

Reflex sympathetic dystrophy (algodystrophy) has commonly been reported after such fractures which develops within the first 9 weeks after injury. The incidence has been reported to be as high as 30% with some individuals remaining symptomatic at the six month stage. It may lead to pain and tenderness of the wrist with finger stiffness and vasomotor disturbances to produce a blue, cold, mottled, painful hand.

Non-union of the radius is almost unheard, of however non-union of the ulnar styloid is relatively common and is most usually painless unless of the hypertrophic non-union type.

The development of post-traumatic osteoarthritis varies from 3 – 18% with a higher incidence in comminuted intra-articular fractures. However, there appears to be a discrepancy between the radiologically apparent changes and symptomatology with only approximately one-third of affected patients being symptomatic.

Median and ulnar nerve compression at the wrist is well described following Colles' fracture and is associated with intra-articular fractures, older age and residual dorsal angulation. The incidence of median nerve compression varies between 0.2% and 17% (mean 2.9%) in the literature. Symptoms may develop many weeks after the fracture has united and may also be associated with increased dorsal angulation. The majority of median nerve compressions require no formal surgical input. Ulnar nerve compression is much less frequent (>1%).

Tendon injuries are uncommon (extensor pollicis longus tendon rupture 0.5% – 1%), with 44–72% occurring in undisplaced fractures and the majority occurring within 9 weeks of injury. Rupture of extensor communis has been described but is very rare.

Mortality does not seem to be higher in patients with Colles' fracture than the general population when co-morbidities are controlled for in the analysis.

Suggested Reading

Cooper C, Atkins E J, Jacobsen S J, O'Fallon W M, Melton L J. (1993) Population-based study of survival after osteoporotic fractures. *Am J Epidemiol* 137(9): 1001–1005.

Koval K J, Zuckerman J D. (1994) Functional recovery after fracture of the hip. *Am J Bone and Joint Surg* 76: 751–756.

Lyons A R. (1997) Clinical outcome and treatment of hip fractures. *JAMA* (In press)

Parker M J, Palmer C R. (1995) Prediction of rehabilitation after hip fracture. *Age Ageing* 24: 96–98.

7

Genes and Osteoporosis

Chris White & John Eisman

Osteoporotic fracture is the clinical endpoint of a lifetime exposure to factors that cause increased skeletal fragility and affects a large population of elderly women and men. Low bone mineral density predicts the risk of an individual sustaining osteoporotic fracture and can be viewed to represent the cumulative exposure over childhood, adolescence and adult years of a number of genetic and environmental factors that affect bone strength. The study of genetic factors in osteoporosis was previously complicated by the fact that fractures occur relatively late in life and, therefore, establishing pedigrees of affected and unaffected members within a family would be logistically complex. However, bone mineral density measurements that predict osteoporotic fracture have allowed the identification of individuals at increased risk of osteoporosis at a younger age. Bone mineral density values provide a quantitative measure of skeletal strength with normally distributed values. Individuals at increased risk of sustaining osteoporotic fracture lie within the lower end of this normal range. This has the advantage of replacing the categorical classification of fracture versus non-fracture with a continuously distributed variable and allows the identification of the degree to which genetic and environmental factors contribute to the variance of this trait. Moreover the identification of genetic factors that determine bone strength must consider the trait in the light of environmental exposure. It is conceivable that genes that predispose to low bone density and fracture in one environment may be protective in a different environment. The study of genetic factors that determine bone strength, therefore, must consider the environment in which the genes are exposed and the context in which those observations are made.

Genetics of Osteoporosis

Osteogenesis Imperfecta as a Discontinuous Trait

Understanding the molecular basis of disorders that lie beyond the clinical and quantifiable normal range has contributed to our understanding of normal bone physiology. Mutations within a number of specific genes have been shown to affect key regulatory and developmental processes in skeletal maturation, turnover and integrity. Thus within a population a small number of individuals and family members sustain fractures that are distinct from the expected clinical presentation and pattern of inheritance evident in the wider population. These distinct clinical entities can be viewed as being discontinuous from the normal population distribution of bone mineral density and expected clinical presentation of osteoporosis and substantial progress has been made in identifying the genetic basis of these disorders. A specific set of gene mutations are responsible for these syndromes that are phenotypically similar and yet occur at an earlier age and/or demonstrate a more classic Mendelian pattern of inheritance with affected and unaffected family members associated with segregating mutations and markers of the disease.

Osteogenesis imperfecta in its various forms presents the model of a discontinuous trait and disease. Mutations within the coding region of Type 1 collagen genes cause osteogenesis imperfecta, with a number of inheritance patterns and degrees of clinical severity that range from spontaneous fractures in utero and childhood years to more mild forms that overlap with the expected pattern of osteoporosis in the wider community. The study of these traits, with earlier onset of disease and identification of affected individuals, has been assisted by the ability to perform classic linkage studies with segregating modes of transmission between generations within families.

Type 1 collagen is the major structural protein in bone and consists of a heterotrimeric complex of two $\alpha 1$ and one $\alpha 2$ molecules. The majority of patients with osteogenesis imperfecta have mutations in the gene for either the pro $\alpha 1$ (I) chain or the pro $\alpha 2$ (I) chain of type I procollagen. The mutant procollagen molecules act in a dominant negative manner. They are incorporated into the type I procollagen molecule that also contains normal pro α chains and cause increased susceptibility to degradation and impaired formation of the extracellular matrix and mineralization. The severity of the clinical phenotype appears to be related to the level of mutant gene expression, the type of mutation and its position within the coding region of the alpha chain. These defects in type I collagen lead to altered skeletal integrity and composition with measurable reductions in bone mineral density, and increased fragility clinically evident as fracture. However these discrete mutations that cause osteogenesis imperfecta affect only a minority of patients within a population. At low frequency they cannot explain the genetic contribution to variability in bone mineral density and the majority of women and men at increased risk of sustaining osteoporotic fractures do not possess these mutations.

Continuous Traits and Quantitative Analysis

Non-invasive techniques for the accurate and reproducible measurement of bone density of the appendicular and axial skeleton allow for the objective evaluation of any genetic influence on this trait. From early childhood to adolescence bone mineral density increases slowly before a pubertal increase in skeletal growth increases bone mass and density towards its peak level. With further aging bone is subsequently lost from this peak level, and bone density at advanced age can be considered a summation of genetic and environmental factors that influence peak bone density and its subsequent loss. Within a population sample men and women of the same age exhibit a wide population variance in bone density with two standard deviations exceeding 20% of the mean bone mineral density value. Part of the variability of bone mineral density is related to age which can be viewed as an index of environments which change significantly over a lifetime.

Variability in a continuous trait such as bone mineral density arises from the multifaceted interaction between changing environments and inherited factors and differs from Mendelian disorders in that heritability does not follow simple segregating modes of transmission. Twin studies provide the opportunity to investigate the relative contribution of genetic and environmental effects to the variability of bone mineral density. While environmental effects such as calcium intake, smoking, alcohol, physical exercise and particularly the menopause are important factors in determining bone mineral density, these studies have identified that genetic factors are the major determinant of bone mineral density, contributing up to 80% of the variance in peak bone mineral density. Moreover genetic factors that determine bone density at different sites within the axial and appendicular skeleton are predominantly shared. However a proportion of specific genetic and environmental effects are operative at sites such as the femoral neck. This would be consistent with unique genes and environmental effects such as exercise and muscle mass influencing osteoporotic fracture risk of the hip. The rate at which bone density changes may also be under genetic control although it is not known whether the same genes that modulate peak bone mass also determine its loss.

Having identified that genetic effects are predominant in determining bone mineral density the quest for specific genes has led to the identification of a number of candidate gene markers that include polymorphisms of the vitamin D receptor and type 1 collagen genes. In comparison to mutations in the coding region of genes causing discontinuous traits such as osteogenesis imperfecta, the majority of the polymorphisms linked to quantifiable continuous traits such as bone density reside within regions that do not code for specific mutations (e.g. promoter, intronic or flanking regions) and the molecular basis for any genetic effect is unknown.

The majority of candidate gene studies have been performed in association studies and have provided conflicting results in different populations as to whether a candidate marker, such as the vitamin D receptor gene polymorphism, is contributing to low bone density and increased osteoporotic fracture risk. 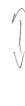 Association studies of a genetic marker with a trait such as low bone mineral density determine whether the marker is over-represented compared to that expected from the frequency of the marker within the population studied. These studies are weakened in the presence of gene-environment interactions, unidentified population admixture or recombination events within populations. A significant gene-environment interaction occurs where genotype determines the physiological response to an environmental variable. Polymorphisms of the vitamin D receptor are related to differences in gut calcium absorption under conditions of dietary calcium restriction which are not present on a replete diet. An analysis of allele frequencies in populations that have inadvertently mixed together, including one population with higher bone density, will lead to the detection of an apparent association between genotype and bone density even when this association does not exist. Recombination between the marker and effect gene could also explain differences between studies in different populations. The polymorphism may be linked to an effect gene distant from the marker in one population that is not evident in other populations because of recombination between the marker and the responsible gene.

Linkage studies provide stronger evidence for a genetic marker contributing to bone density. These studies within families and between sib-pairs provide evidence that inheritance of the marker and the trait are linked. Importantly the ability of these studies to detect a genetic effect depends upon the heritability of the trait, the discordance in bone mineral density between relatives and the number of relationships and markers tested, allele frequency and gene dominance. As a highly heritable trait, bone mineral density is suitable for these quantitative trait analyses but further studies into the genes that influence bone density and osteoporotic fracture risk in the general population will require consideration of the environment in which those observations are made, particularly in relation to those factors already known to influence bone density.

Suggested Reading

Econs MJ, Speer MC. (1996) Genetic studies of complex diseases. *J Bone Miner Res* 11: 1835–40.

Eisman JA. (1996) Vitamin D receptor variants: implications for therapy. *Current Opinions in Genetics and Development* 6: 361–5.

Erlebacher A, Filvaroff EH, Gitelman SE, Derynck R. (1995) Toward a molecular understanding of skeletal development. *Cell* 80: 371–8.

Prockop DJ, Kuivaniemi H, Tromp G. (1994) Molecular basis of osteogenesis imperfecta and related disorders of bone. *Clinics in Plastic Surgery* 21: 407–13.

8

Bone Densitometry, X-Ray and Quantitative Ultrasound

Glen M. Blake & Ignac Fogelman

In the past decade osteoporotic fractures have been recognized as one of the most significant problems in public health. In white women aged 85 years, 95% of fractures of the hip and spine, 80% of forearm fractures and 60% of fractures at other sites are caused by osteoporosis. In the age group 65–84 years the percentages are 90%, 70% and 50% respectively. Increased awareness of the scale of morbidity and mortality attributable to osteoporosis has led to major efforts to develop new treatments aimed at preventing fractures. Alongside these developments there has been rapid evolution of new radiological techniques for the non-invasive assessment of skeletal status.

The technique most associated with the recent rapid growth in clinical applications of bone densitometry is dual X-ray absorptiometry (DXA). DXA was developed in the mid-1980s from the earlier technique of dual photon absorptiometry (DPA) by replacing the ^{153}Gd radionuclide source used in DPA with a X-ray tube. The advantage of DXA is that it allows measurements of bone mineral density (BMD) of the spine and hip with high precision, short scanning times and low radiation dose to the patient. The spine and hip are important measurement sites because they are frequent sites for osteoporotic fractures. Additionally, due to the presence of the metabolically active trabecular bone in the vertebral bodies, the spine is a sensitive site for monitoring response to treatment.

Despite the widespread popularity of DXA scanning of the spine and hip, there is continuing interest in new techniques for assessing the peripheral skeleton. In recent years the old technology of single photon absorptiometry (SPA) used to perform bone densitometry scans of the distal forearm has been updated by replacing the ^{125}I radionuclide source by a X-ray tube. Another new peripheral technique is quantitative ultrasound (QUS) scanning of the calcaneus. Bone ultrasound systems use frequencies in the range 0.1–1.0 MHz and measure broadband ultrasonic attenuation (BUA) and speed of sound (SOS) in the heel. The attraction of QUS devices is that they do not use ionizing radiation. Although DXA is presently the more widely accepted procedure, there is growing evidence that a QUS scan is predictive of fracture risk and is an effective substitute for a BMD measurement in the calcaneus.

Physical Principles of Dual X-Ray Absorptiometry (DXA)

The fundamental principle behind DXA is the measurement of the transmission through the body of X-rays with two different photon energies. Because of the dependence of the attenuation coefficient on atomic number and photon energy, measurement of the transmission factors at two energies enables the areal densities (i.e. mass per unit projected area) of two different types of tissue to be inferred. In DXA scans these are taken to be bone mineral (hydroxyapatite) and soft tissue respectively.

The replacement of the ^{153}Gd radionuclide source used in DPA with a X-ray tube improved the performance of bone densitometers by combining higher photon flux with a smaller diameter source. The availability of an intense, narrow beam of radiation shortened scan times, enhanced image definition, and improved precision. Two alternative methods are used to generate the dual energy X-ray spectrum:

(1) A rare earth filter with a K-absorption edge in the range 40–50 keV splits the X-ray beam into high and low energy components that mimic the emissions from ^{153}Gd. Manufacturers selling DXA systems using this technique include Lunar (Madison, WI), Norland (Fort Atkinson, WI) and Osteometer (Roedovre, Denmark).

(2) Switching the X-ray generator between high and low kVp during alternate half cycles of the mains supply. This method is used by Hologic (Waltham, MA). In Hologic scanners a rotating reference wheel containing bone and soft tissue equivalent filters calibrates the scan image pixel by pixel.

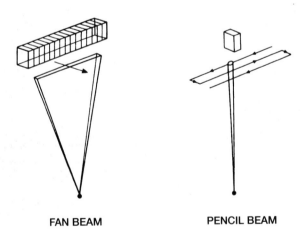

FAN BEAM   PENCIL BEAM

Figure 8.1. Comparison of scanning geometry for a pencil beam DXA system with a single detector (right) and a fan beam scanner with a multidetector array (left).

Fan Beam Dual X-Ray Absorptiometry

The first generation of DXA scanners used a pinhole collimator producing a pencil beam coupled to a single detector in the scanning arm. Since then the most significant development in DXA technology has been the introduction of new systems that use a slit collimator to generate a fan beam coupled to a linear array of detectors (Figure 8.1).

Fan beam studies are acquired by the scanning arm performing a single sweep across the patient instead of the two dimensional raster scan required by pencil beam technology. As a result scan times have been shortened from around 5–10

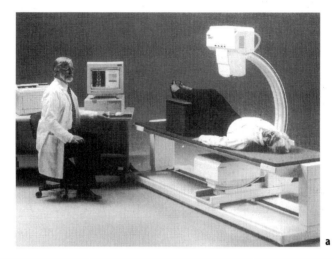

a

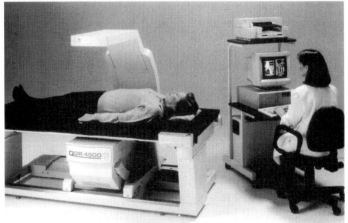

b

Figure 8.2. Illustrations of two advanced DXA systems. (a) The Lunar Expert-XL; (b) The Hologic QDR-4500A.

minutes for early generation scanners to 10–30 seconds for the latest fan beam systems.

In the latest commercial DXA systems such as the Lunar Expert and Hologic QDR-4500 (Figure 8.2) use of a fan beam coupled to a solid-state detector constructed in the form of a multi-element linear array has significantly improved image resolution. This allows easier identification of vertebral structure together with the artifacts due to degenerative disease that can limit DXA studies of the lumbar spine. By supporting the source and detectors on a rotating C-arm, these systems enable lateral scans of the spine to be acquired with the patient in the supine position. With further development this may allow the acquisition of clinically useful vertebral morphometry studies to investigate vertebral fractures.

Dual X-Ray Absorptiometry of the Spine and Hip

Scans of the lumbar spine and hip are the two most frequently performed DXA studies. There are several reasons for this choice, but the most important are the clinical significance of the spine and hip as sites of osteoporotic fractures and the belief that the most reliable indicator of fracture risk at any site is a BMD measurement at that site. Although osteoporosis is a systemic disease, the correlation coefficients between BMD values at different sites are typically around $r \approx 0.7$ and thus a BMD measurement at any one site is far from being a perfect predictor of that at any other site. Therefore individual patients may show unexpectedly low BMD at the femoral neck compared with the lumbar spine and vice-versa. Thus many clinicians believe they can offer more reliable advice to patients about their treatment based on a combination of measurement sites rather than a single site only. The provision of a hip scan alongside a spine scan is particularly helpful in elderly patients in whom spine BMD can be elevated due to degenerative disease and therefore may not reflect true skeletal status.

Another reason for performing BMD scans of the spine is the rapid turnover of the metabolically active trabecular bone in the vertebral bodies which makes the spine the optimum site for monitoring response to treatment. For this reason there is interest in performing DXA scans of the lumbar spine using the lateral instead of the posteroanterior projection since this isolates the vertebral bodies from the posterior elements and better approximates the objective of measuring trabecular bone free of the artifacts caused by degenerative disease. While some studies suggest lateral may be superior to conventional posteroanterior spine DXA for identifying patients with osteopenia and osteoporosis, other studies have reached the opposite conclusion. Thus the diagnostic potential of lateral DXA remains controversial.

Peripheral X-Ray Absorptiometry

Despite the widespread popularity of DXA scanning of the spine and hip, there has been continuing evolution of new instruments for X-ray absorptiometry studies of the peripheral skeleton. In single X-ray absorptiometry (SXA), a low voltage generator (40 kV) replaces the ^{125}I radionuclide source formally used in

SPA. SXA devices require the patient's forearm to be immersed in a water bath while the scan is acquired to correct for the effects of soft-tissue attenuation. The most recent development has been the introduction of peripheral DXA (pDXA) devices based on similar principles to standard DXA equipment. This dispenses with the need for a water bath and allows the patient's forearm to be scanned in air.

The advantages of SXA and pDXA include the small footprint of the devices, relatively low price, and exceptionally low radiation dose. However, although a large number of studies have confirmed the ability of forearm BMD measurements to predict fracture risk, many clinicians prefer to base their advice to patients on spine and hip measurements.

Quantitative Ultrasound Measurements of Bone

The peripheral technique that has raised the most interest in recent years is quantitative ultrasound scanning (QUS) of the calcaneus. Interest in bone ultrasound studies developed following the report of Langton in 1984 that a measurement of broadband ultrasonic attenuation (BUA) in the calcaneus could differentiate between elderly women who had sustained a recent hip fracture and healthy elderly women with no history of fracture. The calcaneus was chosen as the measurement site because it is easily accessible, has a high percentage of trabecular bone, and is weight bearing with a similar pattern of loss as the spine in osteoporosis.

Langton's studies showed that the attenuation coefficient for the propagation of ultrasound through the heel increased linearly with frequency and that, due to the high attenuation in trabecular bone, the frequency range 0.1–1.0 MHz was optimal for determining skeletal status. BUA is defined as the slope of the plot of attenuation against frequency and is measured in units of dB/MHz.

Alongside BUA, most commercial QUS systems also measure the speed of sound (SOS) by dividing the propagation distance by the transit time. The accurate measurement of SOS in bone requires a determination of bone thickness. However, systems that use a water bath for coupling the ultrasound transducers to the patient's heel generally measure the time of flight velocity, defined as the mean velocity of sound through bone, soft-tissue and water. Contact systems using pads that press against the skin measure heel velocity, defined as the mean velocity through bone and soft-tissue. As with BUA, the relatively narrow range of calcaneal widths limits the impact of these different definitions on the clinical utility of the measurements.

A major attraction of bone ultrasound devices is that they do not use ionizing radiation. The instrumentation is less expensive than X-ray technology and the contact systems such as the CUBA (McCue, Winchester, UK) and Sahara (Hologic, Waltham, MA) are highly portable. Therefore ultrasound has a potential for wider applicability than DXA which is largely restricted to major hospital centers.

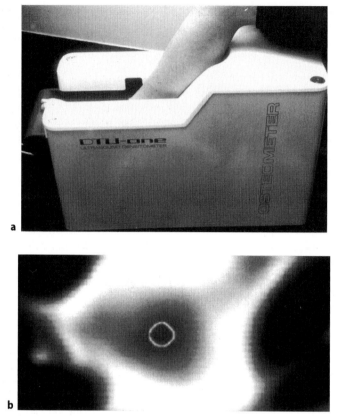

Figure 8.3. (a) Illustration of the Osteometer DTU-one imaging ultrasound system. (b) Scan image of the calcaneus acquired using the DTU-one system.

Most commercial ultrasound systems use a foot support that positions the patient's heel between fixed transducers. Thus the measurement site cannot be adapted to different size and shape of the heel. However, some devices such as the DTU-one (Osteometer, Roedovre, Denmark) produce images of BUA and SOS by performing a raster scan of the calcaneus thus allowing more consistent placement of the measurement site (Figure 8.3).

A widely advocated advantage of QUS is that, because attenuation is largely due to the scattering of sound waves by trabeculae, BUA measurements contain information on the structural integrity of cancellous bone. *In vitro* studies have confirmed that BUA values correlate with histomorphometric parameters of trabecular structure. However, careful mapping of BUA, SOS and BMD in the calcaneus shows such high correlations that, notwithstanding the *in vitro* evidence, there is little variance left to be attributed to structure. This suggests that QUS scans are essentially a substitute for a BMD measurement in the calcaneus.

Future Developments in Dual X-Ray Absorptiometry

DXA scanners have undergone rapid development with the introduction of fan beam systems that have reduced scan times from 5–10 minutes for first generation systems to 10–30 seconds for the latest technology. However, there is a limit to the value of these developments for routine bone densitometry studies. While appointment times have been reduced from around 30 minutes per patient to perhaps 15 minutes, it is difficult to see how patient throughput can be further improved. Moreover, there is little evidence that advances in technology have improved the precision of the BMD measurements, which is a key index of system performance, while radiation dose has tended to increase. There is a case for arguing that simpler and cheaper equipment that made DXA studies more accessible would be of greater benefit to patients.

Future Developments in Quantitative Ultrasound

The current status and future potential of ultrasound techniques have been explored in a recent consensus report. To date, the strongest evidence supporting QUS is the prospective studies of hip fracture predic' on reported in elderly women. Although a strong case can be made that QUS is also expected to predict fracture risk in younger women, more epidemiological studies are required to clarify its role in investigating recently postmenopausal women. A limitation of ultrasound compared with DXA is the relatively poor precision of QUS measurements. This is important because it prevents the use of ultrasound technology in follow-up studies to monitor response to treatment. The problem is compounded by the lack of suitable phantoms for monitoring instrument stability. Notwithstanding these problems, QUS technology has the potential to provide a cheap, portable, radiation free method that will make bone densitometry studies more widely available.

Summary

Over the past decade growing awareness of the impact of osteoporosis on the elderly population and the consequent costs of healthcare has stimulated development of new treatments to prevent fractures together with new imaging technologies to assist in diagnosis. With its ability to perform high precision measurements of the spine and hip, DXA is well suited to meet this latter need. The provision of scanning equipment has expanded rapidly and DXA studies are widely used in diagnosing osteoporosis and aiding decisions over treatment. DXA technology is also playing a major role in clinical research, especially in trials of new treatments. Whether DXA can meet the anticipated need for wider provision of diagnostic services to properly target these treatments is presently unclear. The major alternative is quantitative ultrasound measurements of the calcaneus. Although QUS technology is cheaper than DXA and is proven in its ability to predict fracture risk in the elderly, its future role remains unclear because of poor precision, lack of appropriate phantoms for quality control and doubts about how predict fracture risk in the elderly, its future role remains unclear because of poor precision, lack of appropriate phantoms for quality control and doubts about how to interpret results in younger women. The outcome of this debate will determine the provision of bone densitometry services over the next 10 years.

Suggested Reading

Cummings SR, Black DM, Nevitt MC et al. (1993) Bone density at various sites for prediction of hip fractures. *Lancet* 341: 72–75.

Bauer DC, Glüer C-C, Cauley JA et al. (1997) Broadband ultrasound attenuation predicts fractures strongly and independently of densitometry in older women. *Arch Intern Med* 157: 629–634.

Genant HK, Engelke K, Fuerst T et al. (1996) Noninvasive assessment of bone mineral and structure: state of the art. *J Bone Miner Res* 11: 707–730.

Gregg EW, Kriska AM, Salamone LM et al. (1997) The epidemiology of quanitative ultrasound: a review of the relationships with bone mass, osteoporosis, and fracture risk. *Osteoporosis Int* 7: 89–99.

Wahner HW, Fogelman I. (1994) The Evaluation of Osteoporosis: Dual Energy X-Ray Absorptiometry in Clinical Practice. Martin Dunitz, London.

9

Biochemical Indices and Bone Turnover

Piet Geusens

Biochemical indices are used in the differential diagnosis of osteoporosis and other metabolic bone diseases. In addition to the measurement of parameters of calcium homeostasis (calcium, phosphate, alkaline phosphatase) and the hormones controlling this process (parathyroid hormone, vitamin D metabolites), an increased number of specific markers of bone formation and bone resorption have been developped during recent years.

Biochemical Indices in the Differential Diagnosis of Metabolic Bone Diseases

Several biochemical indices are essential in the differential diagnosis of metabolic bone diseases. These biochemical indices should be measured in case of suspicion of secondary osteoporosis. In Table 9.1 some examples of this additional information in the differential diagnosis of osteoporosis and other metabolic bone diseases are given.

Assessment of the Level of Bone Turnover

The assessment of the level of bone turnover has markedly improved with the development of sensitive and specific biochemical markers in the circulation and urine reflecting the level of bone formation and bone resorption (Table 9.2).

These biochemical indices of skeletal metabolism are valuable in the study of osteoporosis and have contributed to our understanding the pathophysiology of osteoporosis and the effects of treatment in group studies. At the time of the menopause, the biochemical indices of bone turnover increase markedly in the order of 30-100% and decrease after treatment with antiresorptive agents such as hormonal replacement therapy. Prospective clinical studies suggest a relation between parameters of bone turnover, bone loss and fracture risk. In some instances, the combination of bone mass measurements with parameters of bone turnover could better predict subgroups of patients at risk for accelerated bone loss. Bone markers are therefore likely to play an important role in the management of osteoporosis. A combination of markers for bone formation and resorption might reflect the different different events of the complex process of bone remodeling, but the optimal combination which may influence therapy has not been yet defined.

Table 9.1. Biochemical indices in the differential diagnosis of osteoporosis. Some examples of the value in differential diagnosis are shown.

Measurement	Change	Differential diagnosis
Calcium		
- serum	↑	increased bone resorption (e.g. hyperparathyroidism, bone metastasis, myeloma)
	↓	parathyroid hypofunction or hyporesponsiveness, osteomalacia
- urine	↑	hypercalciuria (drugs, hyperabsorption from the gut, renal loss)
Phosphate		
- serum	↓	hyperparathyroidism, heredetary or acquired osteomalacia
- urine	↑	phosphate diabetes
Total alkaline phosphatase	↑	Paget's disease, hyperparathyroidism, osteomalacia, fracture, renal osteodystrophy, liver disease
	↓	hypophosphatasia
Immunoreactive parathyroid hormone (iPTH)	↑	hyperparathyroidism (primary, secondary)
	↓	hypoparathyroidism
Vitamin D metabolites		
- 25 (OH) D_3	↓	deficiency (diet, sun)
Indices of bone turnover		see Table 9.2
- formation	↑	
- resorption	↑	

The use of measurements of bone turnover in daily clinical practice in the individual patient is essential in the diagnosis and monitoring of diseases such as Paget's disease and tumor-induced osteolysis. However, in the evaluation of the patient with osteoporosis, the interpretation is hampered by the high intra- and inter-individual variations of these parameters. Indices of bone turnover show seasonal and circadian variations. Therefore, the use in osteoporosis is limited and studies are currently performed to further evaluate the place of bone turnover parameters in the diagnosis and treatment of osteoporosis in the individual patient.

Table 9.2. Biochemical indices of bone turnover in osteoporosis.

	Source	Measurement in
Formation		
Total alkaline phosphatase	liver – bone – gut	serum
Bone-specific alkaline phosphatases	osteoblasts	serum
Osteocalcin	osteoblasts	serum
Procollagen peptides	osteoblasts	urine
Resorption		
Urinary calcium/creatinine	bone – kidney – other organs	urine
Tartrate-resistant acid phosphatase	osteoclasts – prostate – blood cells	serum
Hydroxyproline	collagen degradation in bone – skin – liver	urine
Hydroxyline glycosides	collagen degradation in bone – skin – liver	urine
Pyridinium crosslinks (pyridinoline, deoxypyridinoline) and related peptides	collagen cross-links in bone	urine, serum?

Suggested reading

Delmas PD. (1988) Biochemical markers of bone turnover in osteoporosis. In: Riggs BL, Melton LJ (eds.) *Osteoporosis: Etiology, Diagnosis and Management.* Raven Press, NewYork.

Stepan JJ, Pospichal J, Presl J et al. (1987) Bone loss and biochemical indices of bone remodeling in surgical induced posymenopausal women. *Bone* 8: 279–284.

Eastell R, Hampton L, Colwell A. (1990) Urinary collagen crosslinks are highly correlated with radio-isotopic measurtements of bone resorption. In: Christiansen C, Overgaard K (eds.) *Proceedings of the Third International Symposium on Osteoporosis.* Osteopress, Aalborg, pp. 469–470.

Eastell R, Calvo MS, Burritt MF, Offord KP, Russell RGG. (1992) Anormalities in circadian patterns of bone resorption and renal calcium conservation in type I osteoporosis. *J Clin Endocrinol Metab* 74:487–494.

Hansen MA, Kirsten O, Riis BJ, Christiansen C. (1991) Role of peak bone mass and bone loss in postmenopausal osteoporosis: 12 year study. *BMJ* 303:961–964.

10

Extraskeletal Risk and Protective Factors for Fractures

Jan Dequeker & Steven Boonen

Although there are general risk factors for all types of fragility fractures, the risk may differ according to the type of fracture and the period of life when these fractures occur.

Two types of fractures are commonly distinguished: type I fractures occurring at trabecular bone sites, particularly at the spine and the forearm distal radius, affecting women six times more than men in the age of 50 to 65 years; type II fractures occurring at more cortical bone sites, in particular the proximal femur and the humerus and other long bones, affecting women two times more than men from the age of 70 years onwards. The pathophysiology behind each of these types is different. Type I osteoporosis is related to hormonal changes, in particular sex hormones and corticosteroids, while type II osteoporosis is related to aging and general fragility.

Risk Factors – General Aspects

In both types of fragility fractures additional factors have exerted for long periods a silent negative or positive effect on the bone reserves. Some of them are modifiable and others are not (Table 10.1). Among the modifiable factors corticosteroids play an important and strategic role.

Although at present, the best risk factor estimation for osteoporosis is the measurement of bone density in particularly by DEXA spine or hip, clinical risk factors estimates should not be disregarded. Low bone density is only one of a number of the risk factors for fracture in menopausal women, some of which have similar independent estimates for risk association with fractures. These include a history of maternal hip fracture, previous fractures of any type after the age of 50, self-rated health as fair to poor, previous hyperthyroidism, inability to rise from a chair without using one's arms, a faster resting pulse rate, and poorer depth perception.

An important new concept has recently emerged concerning risk factors for osteoporosis. Each risk factor on its own, although related to osteoporosis, is not sensitive and specific for detection of the patient with a low bone density and at high risk for fracture. But a combination of several risk factors is much more sensitive and helpful for identification of patients at risk for osteoporosis and to assist in clinical decision making to prevent osteoporosis or to prevent further fractures at any age or period in life.

Table 10.1. Risk factors for osteoporosis according to pathophysiologic background.

Background	Factor
Genetic	Family history of osteoporotic fracture Caucasians-Asians > Blacks Absence of generalized osteoarthritis
Anthropometric	Small stature Fair, thin, pale skinned Thin body habitus Long hip axis length
Hormonal	Women > men Early menopause Late menarche Nulliparity Exercise-induced amenorrhea Anorexia nervosa
Dietary	Low dietary calcium Excess protein Excessive alcohol
Lifestyle	Sedentary Smoking
Concurrent illness and drugs	Gastrectomy, hyperparathyroidism Rheumatoid arthritis Hyperthyroidism Cushing's syndrome, corticosteroid therapy Neurological diseases: cerebrovascular accident, Parkinson's disease, dementia Transplantation

The National Osteoporosis Foundation of the United States uses a combination of the following risk factors: smoking, a maternal fracture history and low body weight. Individuals with more than two of these risk factors have a greater than 30% increase in fracture risk at any age.

Risk Factors More Specific for Hip Fracture

Low Body Mass Index

Both low body weight and low body mass index have been documented to increase the risk of hip fracture, even after adjustment for bone mineral density. This relationship may be partially due to an underlying, confounding correspondence between body weight and bone mass as a result of enhanced conversion of androgens to estrogens in peripheral fat. However, low body mass index may also be associated with increased loads applied to the femur due to insufficient absorption of impact energy in soft tissues.

Previous Fractures

Several prospective studies have indicated that previous fractures of the proximal femur, the distal radius and the proximal humerus increase the risk of sustaining a subsequent fracture of the hip. Moreover, a woman whose mother had a hip fracture, especially before the age of 80, is at least twice as likely to have a hip fracture herself as a woman without such a maternal history. Other types of maternal fractures, on the other hand, do not increase hip fracture risk, and the risk is independent of bone mass, height, and weight. Inherited characteristics of the proximal femur besides density, or perhaps a propensity to fall on the hip, may account for this familial predisposition.

Medical Conditions

The onset of a fall initiates several types of protective responses which may attenuate the force of impact and decrease the risk of a fracture. As the effectiveness of these responses depends on muscle function, the decline in muscle strength that occurs with age might impair protective responses of elderly fallers. Consistent with this assumption, *muscle weakness* has been shown to be associated with the risk for hip fracture. In addition to neuromuscular dysfunction, poor visual functioning is likely to increase the risk of falls in general and to impair the protective responses when a fall occurs. Numerous studies have indeed indicated that *impaired vision* increases the risk of hip fracture. According to recent prospective evidence, poor depth perception and a reduced ability to perceive contrast may be particularly important, rather than impaired visual acuity. Similarly, fracture risk is also elevated in patients with *cognitive impairment*. Except for being associated with compromised protective responses, cognitive impairment may be associated with fracture risk because impaired judgment may predispose cognitively impaired persons to engage in more hazardous activities.

Both thyroxine and triiodothyronine directly stimulate bone resorption, and the effect is dose-dependent. One consequence is an increase in bone turnover seen consistently with *hyperthyroidism*. The increase in bone resorption is not fully compensated for by an increase in bone formation, resulting in net bone loss. Clinically, this imbalance between bone formation and resorption is reflected by a strong association between hyperthyroidism and the risk of hip fracture. Deleterious effects of *primary hyperparathyroidism* on the skeleton have also been demonstrated in numerous studies, particularly at sites with a predominance of cortical bone. However, a recent population-based, prospective study did not show an increase in hip fracture risk in primary hyperparathyroidism. Finally, cross-sectional data have suggested an increase in hip fracture risk with non-insulin-dependent *diabetes mellitus*, but these estimates were based on very small numbers. Moreover, almost all studies indicate that bone mass is unaffected by diabetes, and diabetes was not associated with an increased risk of hip fracture in a recent prospective study among women 65 years of age or older.

Low Vitamin D Status

A low vitamin D status (lack of sun exposure, low vitamin D diet) in frail elderly living indoors for months or years, is associated with increased incidence of hip fracture. Vitamin D deficiency in addition to renal insufficiency induces muscle weakness and secondary hyperparathyroidism.

Medications

Studies of bone mineral density at different sites, including the proximal femur, have indicated a significant loss of bone during *corticosteroid therapy*. There is evidence that steroid-induced bone loss at the hip is most marked during the initial months of therapy, with subsequent slowing. It is not known if there is a threshold dose for corticosteroid effect, but bone loss has been consistently documented with doses exceeding 7.5 mg of prednisone per day. In line with these densitometric data, case-controlled studies have provided evidence to suggest that the use of steroids is associated with an increase in incidence of hip fractures.

Nonsteroidal drugs have also been implied in the pathogenesis of fractures of the proximal femur in elderly women. In particular, the use of *psychotropic drugs* has been hypothesized to increase the risk of hip fractures by increasing the likelihood of falls or by increasing the proportion of falls that result in a fracture. Both cross-sectional and prospective studies have indeed shown that the use of long-acting benzodiazepines is associated with an increased risk of hip fracture. By contrast, no association is observed with the use of short half-life drugs.

Physical Inactivity

In several case-controlled studies, customary physical inactivity was found to be an independent risk factor for hip fracture in elderly people. In accordance with these cross-sectional reports, recent prospective data have confirmed that decreased levels of physical activity are associated with a substantially increased risk of hip fracture. The protective effect of physical activity may partially be accounted for by an increase in muscle strength, but physical inactivity remains strongly associated with hip fracture risk after adjusting for test results on neuromuscular function. Similarly, the detrimental effect of physical inactivity may be complicated by the presence of underlying chronic diseases which may confound the physical inactivity-fracture risk relationship. However, the relationship is unaffected by adjustment for dependence in daily living activities, a marker of general disability.

Caffeine Intake, Smoking, and Alcohol Consumption

Several cohort studies have provided evidence that *caffeine consumption* increases the risk of hip fracture. Adjustment for bone density does not substantially affect the risk of hip fracture associated with caffeine intake, suggesting that caffeine may influence the risk of fracture in other ways.

Cross-sectional as well as longitudinal data have provided evidence that *smoking* adversely affects bone density and increases the rate of bone loss at a variety of skeletal sites, including the proximal femur. In line with these densitometric data, current smoking was found to be associated with an increased risk of hip fracture, both in case-controlled and most (but not all) prospective population-based studies. The exact mechanism for this association has not been established yet, but may be mediated through an effect of smoking on estrogen metabolism and calcium absorption. In addition, smokers differ from their non-smoking counterparts in several potentially important respects including a lower body mass index and a lower degree of physical activity.

Current *alcohol intake* has generally been found to increase the risk of hip fracture in women aged less than 65 years. Both deleterious effects on bone metabolism and an increased risk of trauma have been implied in the pathogenesis of alcohol-related fractures. In elderly women, however, several cross-sectional and longitudinal studies failed to find a positive association between moderate alcohol intake and risk of hip fracture, suggesting that the effect may be confined to younger people.

Protective Factors

Obesity and Osteoarthritis

Clinical observations in patients who have symptomatic osteoporosis have revealed that patients with vertebral collapse and hip fracture have a lower than average body weight, less subcutaneous fat, a thin body habitus and rarely suffer from generalized osteoarthritis. Obese women have a greater load and thus have increased mechanical forces on the bones which are beneficial. In addition to these increased mechanical forces, subcutaneous fat plays an important role after the menopause, when the only source of female hormone estrogen comes from the conversion – also called aromatization – of androstenedione (a male related hormone) into oestrone by subcutaneous fat.

Osteoarthritis protects against osteoporosis as large epidemiological studies have shown that cases with mild or severe osteoarthritis have a 10% higher bone density at all measured sites, corrected for osteophytes and body weight, and this increase corresponds to 10 years of hormone replacement therapy or 10 kg of extra body weight.

The inverse relationship between osteoarthritis and osteoporosis is of particular interest because osteoarthritis affects about two thirds of the elderly population and therefore osteoarthritis could eventually be a good help to select patients for preventive therapy against osteoporosis. Because the first clinical signs of generalized osteoarthritis become apparent around the age of 50 in the form of Heberden or Bouchard nodes at the finger joints, respectively at the distal and proximal interphalangeal finger joints, these observations gain in importance and may help the clinician to decide about long-term prophylaxis of osteoporosis. Although osteoarthritis protects against osteoporosis, this does not mean that osteoarthritis cases will never sustain a fracture. Osteoarthritis, however, may postpone the occurrence of fragility fractures for a number of years.

A larger bone density in osteoarthritis is most likely genetically determined. The alteration in bone characteristics in osteoarthritis is not restricted to quantitative elements as increased bone density and bone mass, but also to qualitative elements as shown by a change in bone composition and repair.

Summary

Although the best risk factor estimation for osteoporosis is the measurement of bone density, estimation of clinical risk factors and protective factors should not be disregarded. A combination of several risk factors is much more sensitive and helpful to identify patients at risk for osteoporosis and to assist in clinical decision making. Protective factors such as obesity and osteoarthritis on the other hand may help to identify patients not at high risk for osteoporosis.

11

Dual Energy X-Ray Absorptiometry in Daily Clinical Practice

Piet Geusens

Indications for Bone Mass Measurements

There is a growing consensus on the indications for bone mass measurements in clinical practice. As bone mass measurements predict a patient's risk of fracture, there is international agreement between experts that osteoporosis can be diagnosed on the basis of bone mass measurements, even in the absence of prevalent fractures and that bone mass measurements provide information that can affect the patient's management. The choice of the appropriate measurement site(s) for the assessment of fracture risk may vary depending on specific medical circumstances of the patient and should in any given clinical circumstance be based on an understanding of the strength and limitations of the different techniques. Furthermore, bone mass data should be accompanied by a clinical interpretation.

Table 11.1. Clinical indications for bone densitometry.

Presence of strong risk factors:	premature menopause (<45 years)
	prolonged secondary amenorrhoea
	primary hypogonadism
	anorexia nervosa
	malabsorption
	primary hyperparathyroidism
	long-term corticosteroid therapy
	organ transplantation
	chronic renal failure
	myelomatosis
	hyperthyroidism
	prolonged immobilization
Previous fracture of hip, spine, or wrist	
Radiological evidence of osteopenia or vertebral abnormality	
Monitoring:	bone loss ('fast losers')
	treatment effect (non-responders)

Indications for bone mass measurements are given in Table 11.1. In contrast to these well documented indications it is recognized that there are currently insufficient data to justify convincingly the use of bone mass measurements to screen unselected people. Bone mass measurements that will not be followed by appropriate evaluation, or that will not influence the patients' or physicians' behavior, are not advisable.

Interpretation of Bone Mass Measurements

For interpretation of bone densitometry results, a value of bone density is mostly reported in terms of differences in standard deviations from the mean of age- and sex-matched controls ('Z-score') or to the mean peak bone density ('T-score'). From a practical point of view, this scoring method is preferred over comparisons in percent, as percent differences from the mean can only be well interpreted when the normal variation in the population is taken into account. It is important to distinguish fracture risk assessment as a prognostic tool from the diagnosis of osteoporosis as a diagnostic tool.

A working group of the World Health Organization has recently proposed several diagnostic categories on the basis of the results of the T-score of bone densitometry (Figure 11.1).

(1) *Normal bone density*: bone density within 1 standard deviation (SD) of the young adult reference mean

(2) *Osteopenia*: bone density more than 1 SD below the young adult mean but less than 2.5 SD below this value

(3) *Osteoporosis*: bone density 2.5 SD or more below the young adult mean

(4) *Severe ('established') osteoporosis*: bone density more than 2.5 SD below the young adult mean in the presence of one or more fragility fractures.

Using this definition of osteoporosis, 30% of postmenopausal women have

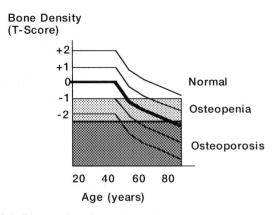

Figure 11.1. Diagnostic categories on the basis of the results of the T-score of bone densitometry (World Health Organization).

osteoporosis and more than 50% had already a fragility fracture. These diagnostic criteria are a basis for appropriate diagnosis and can be helpful in decisions on prevention and treatment. These criteria are likely to change as experience increases, such as for the definition of hypertension. However, they provide a framework for clinical practice and further investigation, and permit greater accuracy in describing the extent and the characteristics of osteoporosis.

For the final interpretation of bone densitometry, quality control procedures and an appropriate protocol are needed. Quality control depends on regular calibration, the use of adequate reference ranges, positioning of the patient, definition of regions of interest and exclusion of interfering factors, such as extraskeletal calcifications.

Examples of protocols lay-outs for bone densitometry are shown in Figure 11.2 (lumbar spine) and Figure 11.3 (hip).

Bone Measurements for Monitoring Progress

In longitudinal studies precision is more important. Precision is generally better *in vitro* than *in vivo* and better in younger than in elderly or osteoporotic patients. In the clinical setting, the precision of photon absorptiometry (1–4%) – and this is true for all other current techniques – is insufficient to measure short-term changes of the order of 1–5% per year in individual patients. Since the abnormal

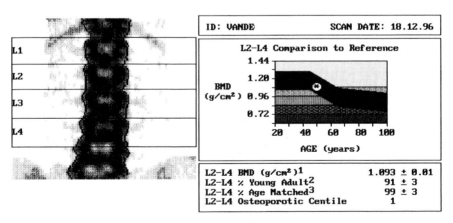

Figure 11.2. Results of bone densitometry in the lumbar spine (Lunar device as an example).

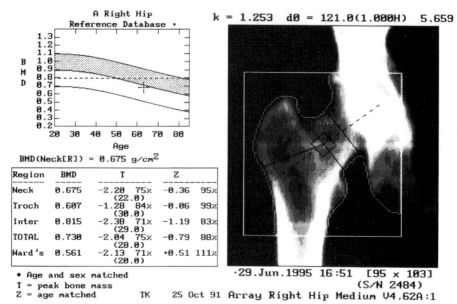

Figure 11.3. Results of bone densitometry in the hip (Hologic device as an example).

bone loss and any therapeutic response are both slow and low (1–5 % per year), changes in a particular individual over a span of a few months or even a full year cannot be detected within acceptable confidence limits. In group studies however, the rates of loss as indicators of therapeutic effect can be evaluated over a shorter period because reproducibility errors will be damped by the larger numbers involved. For monitoring metabolic bone diseases and their response to treatment, bone mass measurements should be performed at a skeletal site containing predominantly trabecular bone and at another one with predominantly cortical bone.

Global Risk Assessment for Osteoporosis

In Chapters 5 and 10, it has been shown that global fracture risk in an individual patient is dependent on skeletal and extra-skeletal factors. A systematic screening for clinical risk factors is possible in daily practice. Furthermore, bone densitometry should be performed when a greater clinical risk for osteoporosis is present, especially when the result of the bone densitometry will affect treatment. When performing risk assessment, special attention is required for identifying reversible (e.g. low bone density, impaired vision) or expected risk factors (e.g. bone loss early after menopause, corticosteroid therapy). As an example, some typical clinical circumstances for risk assessment for osteoporosis are depicted in Table 11.2.

Table 11.2. Some examples of typical clinical circumstances involved in risk assessment for osteoporosis. Clinical cases in 4 women and in 1 man are shown and should be read from top to bottom. For specifications of risk factors, see Chapters 5 and 10. (+ = Yes, − = No).

Risk assessment	Women				Man
History					
Personal					
− age	50	65	65	85	65
− hypogonadism	+	+	+	+	−
− diseases	−	−	−	+	Chronic bronchitis
− medication	−	−	−	+	Steroids
− life style					
smoking	−	−	−	−	+
alcohol	−	−	−	−	+
physical activity	+	−	+	−	−
diet					
− calcium	+	+	+	−	−
− protein	+	+	+	−	−
− vitamin D	+	−	+	−	+
− previous falls	−	+	−	+	−
− previous fracture	−	+	−	+	−
− institutionalized	−	−	−	+	−
Familial					
− hip fracture in the mother	−	+	−	+	−
− cardiovascular disease	+	−	−	−	−
Clinical examination					
− body mass index	low	nl	high	low	nl
− race (Caucasian)	+	+	+	+	+
− muscle strength	nl	nl	nl	low	low
− balance, gait	nl	nl	nl	bad	nl
− vision	nl	bad	nl	bad	nl
Biochemical evaluation					
− suspicion of secondary osteoporosis	no	yes	no	yes	yes
− 'fast loser'	+	−	−	+	+
Bone densitometry					
− T-score	nl	low	nl	low	low
Risk for osteoporotic fractures	low	high	low	high	high

Summary

Measurement of bone mass has largely contributed to our understanding of age-related bone growth, bone loss and osteoporosis. Several measurement techniques are now available. Taking into account the accuracy and precision in normal and pathological conditions, these methods are a valuable diagnostic tool in daily clinical practice for diagnosis and follow-up of the individual patient. They should be interpreted together with the global risk assessment in each patient.

Suggested Reading

Consensus Development Statement: Who are candidates for prevention and treatment for osteoporosis? (1997) *Osteoporosis Int* 7: 1–6.

Consensus of an international panel on the clinical utility of bone mass measurements in the detection of low bone mass in the adult population. (1996) *Calcif Tiss Int* 58: 207–214.

Genant HK et al. (1996) Noninvasive assessment of bone mineral and structure: state of the art. *J Bone Miner Res* 11: 707–730.

Johnston CC Jr, Melton LJ III, Lindsay R, Eddy DM. (1989) Clinical indications for bone mass measurements: report from the Scientific Advisory Board of the National Osteoporosis Foundation. *J Bone Miner Res* 4(Suppl. 2): 1–28.

Kanis JA, Melton LJ, Christiansen C, Johnston CC, Khaltev N. (1994) The diagnosis of osteoporosis. *J Bone Miner Res* 9: 1137–41.

Ross PD, Heilbrun LK, Wasnich RD, Davis JW, Vogel JM. (1989) Perspectives: methodologic issues in evaluating risk factors for osteoporotic fractures. *J Bone Miner Res* 4: 649–56.

12

Differential Diagnosis: Back Pain and Osteoporosis

Maren G. Scholz & Helmut W. Minne

Back pain is very common in industrial countries. In Europe and the USA the lifetime prevalence is 60%, and 35% of the population suffer from back pain at least once a year. The incidence of back pain in elderly people is even higher than this. The causes of back pain are considered to be multifactorial and in explaining the high incidence rates, osteoporotic fractures appear not to be considered as important as chronic musculoligamentous strain, osteoarthritis, chronic intervertebral disc disease, facet joints and spinal stenosis. However, pain is still one of the most limiting symptoms for osteoporosis patients.

Osteoporosis in a progressive stage leads to the destruction of the structure and function of the bone. As a result fractures occur. In the spine the regions T7-T9 and T12-L1 are especially at risk because of the natural kyphotic shape and the resulting forces on the vertebrae. Incident fractures often entail acute severe pain for several months. Consecutive vertebral fractures and subsequent malfunction of joints, tendons and muscles can cause chronic pain. Fractures are often associated with chronic pain perception, both in clinical practice and in research approaches. For instance, when a physician looks at an x-ray which shows multiple fractures patients will often hear: "you must be in terrible pain". However there is a great variability in patients' pain perception with a comparable degree of somatic lesion.

There is no specific pain pattern which can be attributed to osteoporosis. When comparing patients with osteoporosis and chronic low back pain due to other causes, it has been found that although pain is the leading symptom in both groups there are no differences in intensity and frequency. Osteoporosis related pain perception seems to be more localized in the thoracic spine as opposed to back pain which occurs in the lower back due to other causes such as chronic disc degeneration or osteoarthritis. It is also assumed that pain which occurs from a recent fracture is usually felt in the region where the fracture occurs. However drawing any definite conclusion about location and pattern is still not possible.

Osteoporosis is often described as "the silent thief". Patients who are suffering from this disease do not know that they are – as long as no fractures will occur. It is not yet possible to make any firm statement about whether osteopenia can produce back pain as a result of microtraumatic lesions or from static changes in the bone structure. At this time most research denies any relation between low bone mass and high pain perception.

Half of the spinal fractures are asymptomatic. Some 30 to 50% of patients attribute the pain arising from a fracture incident to other problems of the back. But when asked about the attendant circumstances about 80% of the patients can give further details. Study results show that only 35% of the fractures which are detectable on x-rays are clinically diagnosed. This further indicates that fractures can be easily overlooked in clinical practice. However symptoms such as a high degree of kyphosis and height loss over 4 cm suggest the presence of at least one fracture in the vertebral column.

As described above, there are several difficulties which impede a deeper understanding of the relationship between vertebral lesion and quality of life parameters such as pain. A further complicating factor is the fact that there is no gold standard for the assessment of these two parameters. The number of fractures or deformities discovered is dependent on investigator, method and model: different methodological approaches can produce a great variation in incidence and prevalence of fractures that are found. Measurements of pain are equally problematic. The results of questionnaires that inquire about the pain that patients suffer are biased by the great differences in the way that pain is perceived whereas physical pain measurements do not take the patients' sensual and emotional differences into consideration. It therefore comes as no surprise that such ill-defined and differing investigation methods produce results on the relations between back pain and osteoporotic lesion which create more confusion than clarification.

In spite of all these limitations, some consensus exists about the relation between vertebral deformities and back pain:

- Patients with vertebral fractures experience reinforcement of pain during physical activity. Bending, standing, rising from lying and doing housework all aggravate the pain. Relief of pain tends to occur with rest, physiotherapy, heat applications and moving around.
- Strong correlations have been shown between vertebral deformities and clinical symptoms. However, the number of fractures is a poor predictor for the limitations in daily living, pain and other quality of life parameters. Continual measurements of spine deformity are better suited to explaining the relation between the lesion and the pain than the number of fractures.
- The relationship between deformities and pain is not linear, but there is a significant relation between clinical measures of spinal deformation (such as height loss, distance from occiput to wall as an approximation for kyphosis and distance from iliac to ribs) and pain perception. Patients with stooped back and a height loss over 4 cm are twice as likely to experience pain than those without these clinical symptoms. Chronic pain in patients with osteoporosis is related to a high degree of kyphosis. Indeed, biomechanical stresses produced by excessive curvature of the thoracic spine are believed to be a common cause of chronic back pain. Compensatory hyperlordosis in the lumbar spine could cause chronic low back pain too, but our clinical

experience shows only few patients with kyphosis where compensatory lordosis is present. Static changes, for example extended kyphosis, cannot exclusively be explained by vertebral deformation. There is for example an age-related increase of 6% or higher per decade in kyphosis index independent from specific diseases. Various techniques have been used to quantify thoracic curvature (Debrunner kyphometer, body contour index, distance from occiput to wall). Despite measurement problems, it seems appropriate to measure kyphotic deformity as a means for getting a further insight into individual pain perception.

Therefore, we can conclude that fractures are associated with height loss and kyphosis and are related to an increased risk of pain and disability.

A large cross-sectional study in 2992 women indicated that the degree of deformity for each vertebral body explains pain perception better than the number of fractures or deformities. Each woman's worst vertebral deformity was correlated to back pain and disabilities in daily living. Women with vertebral deformities below 4 SD show no correlation to these parameters whereas women whose deformity was greater or equal to 4 SD had a 1.9 times higher risk of moderate to severe back pain, a 2.6 times higher risk of disability and were 2.5 times more likely to loose more than 4 cm in height. There was no increase in this relative risk when multiple fractures below 4 SD were assessed but multiple fractures greater or equal to 4 SD seemed to enhance the relative risk of pain and disabilities even more.

It has been found that one incident fracture during the last 4 years causes a 2.8 times higher risk for pain, two recent fractures cause a 7.8 times higher risk for pain and three incident fractures increase the risk of pain by 21.7 times. The risk of disability also rises (relative risk: 4.0) with a recent fracture. It is difficult to define the cut-off when a fracture is recent or old. However data indicate that a fracture older than 2 years is less painful and less distressing than a recent fracture.

In order to explain the great differences in pain, it is insufficient to concentrate only on somatic factors. Other factors seem to play a major role in this context. Psychosocial aspects are also relevant for explaining pain perception. Individual differences and capabilities are linked to the perception of chronic pain and social factors (such as social support) also have an impact. The lack of Sense of Coherence (SOC), for example, which is the capability of a person to realize comprehensibility, manageability and meaningfulness in his or her own life is associated with pain. It is higher in the low pain groups than in the groups with severe pain. SOC itself is not independent from social aspects (such as marital status and net income) and the number of critical life events. Patients with high pain perception also show a higher depression score. These results indicate that it might be possible to reduce pain and improve quality of life with adequate psychological intervention models which focus on improving SOC and reducing depression as an additional necessity to the conventional drug and functional therapy.

In conclusion, back pain is one of the leading symptoms in patients with osteoporosis but there is no causal linking between somatic lesion and individual pain perception.

Suggested Reading

Cummings S, Tabor H. (1995) The epidemiology of vertebral fractures. In: Genant H, Jergas M, v. Kujik C. (eds) *Vertebral Fracture in Osteoporosis*, pp. 3–14.

Ettinger B, Black D, Nevitt M et al. (1992) Contribution of vertebral deformities to chronic back pain and disability. *J Bone Miner Res* 7(4): 449–455.

Ettinger B, Cooper C. (1995) Clinical assessment of vertebral fractures. In: Genant H, Jergas M, v. Kujik C. (eds) *Vertebral Fracture in Osteoporosis,* pp. 15–19.

Huang C, Ross P, Wasnich R. (1996) Vertebral fractures and other predictors of back pain among older women. *J Bone Miner Res* 11(7): 1026–1032.

Leidig-Bruckner G et al. (1997) Clinical grading of spinal osteoporosis. Quality of life components and spinal deformity in women with chronic low back pain and women with vertebral osteoporosis. *J Bone Miner Res* 12(4): 1–13.

Leidig G, Minne HW, Sauer P et al. (1990) A study of complaints and their relation to vertebral destruction in patients with osteoporosis. *Bone and Mineral* 8: 217–229.

13

Differential Diagnosis: Bone Pain and Fractures

Carlo Gennari

Bone pain is a very common feature of many metabolic bone diseases such as metastatic bone disease, osteoporosis and Paget's disease of bone. The bone pain that accompanies such diseases can very often be severe and debilitating. Attempts to relieve pain in these conditions can dominate the management of the overall disease. A common factor in many metabolic bone diseases is increased bone resorption, mediated by activated osteoclasts, a pathophysiological process that often results in pain by a variety of direct and indirect mechanisms. The mechanism of pain is complex and depends on an increasing number of interrelated pathways and mediators. The sensation of pain from bone is still poorly understood, although it is believed to depend mainly on the action of nociceptors in the periosteum and around joint surfaces, whilst areas such as the cortex and bone marrow are believed to be insensitive to pain. In general terms bone pain can be categorized as arising from one of the following mechanisms: a direct action on bone nociceptors or a secondary mechanical effect. A number of chemical mediators can directly affect bone nociceptors, in addition to structural damage to nerve fibres by direct compression of tissue. Often mechanical pressures on an area of bone that is pain insensitive may alter the shape of a nearby joint and cause pain. For instance, a vertebral compression fracture may distort a nearby apophyseal joint, triggering nociceptors and resulting in pain. Although the mechanisms of bone pain, in a variety of different diseases, may have common pathways, the role of certain mediators in the cause of the pain may differ and this may have therapeutic implications.

There is little evidence that bone loss itself causes symptoms, until such time that a fracture occurs; even a vertebral fracture can remain asymptomatic. It is perhaps this clinically silent nature of the disease that makes osteoporosis such a challenge. Therefore, in osteoporosis, all the clinical manifestations are a direct or indirect consequence of fracture and thus, bone pain is the main clinical symptom.

There are both osseous and extra-osseous factors that contribute to fracture in patients with osteoporosis: the osseous factors include decreased skeletal mass, altered architectural orientation of skeletal structures and reduced strength of the skeletal material. The extra-osseous factors include principally propensity to fall, poor reflex response to a fall, inadequate energy absorption by soft tissue at the point of impact. The relative contribution of each factor will vary from person to person as well as across the different fracture syndromes. Often decreased mass is considered the single most important factor in most patients, but this may be because we have recognized it the longest and understand it the best.

In clinical practice non-specific back pain is a very common complaint, the causes of which are extremely varied. In general, osteoporosis is not associated with back pain until a vertebral fracture has occurred. Even when a fracture has occurred, many patients are without obvious clinical symptoms. Osteoporotic vertebral fracture should always be considered within the differential diagnosis of any non-specific back pain. There are many major diseases that cause bone pain (Table 13.1).

Table 13.1. Diseases causing bone pain.

Trauma or osteoporotic fracture	
Osteomalacia:	Vitamin D deficiency
	Anticonvulsants
	Renal failure
	Hypophosphataemia
	Acidosis (systemic or renal tubular)
	Intoxication (bisphosphonates, fluoride, aluminium)
Myeloma	
Metastatic malignancy	
Paget's disease of bone	
Osteomyelitis	
Hyperparathyroidism	
Fibrous dysplasia	
Osteogenesis imperfecta	
Pseudo-bone pain:	Polymyalgia rheumatica
	Parkinsonism
	Hypothyroidism

The importance of reaching the correct diagnosis is self evident, as some of the causes are invariably fatal and others may be easily treated or are fatal if left untreated. The most common causes of true bone pain, as opposed to joint pain, are trauma, osteoporosis and malignancy. Distinguishing among these different causes can be difficult and some diagnoses are often only made after exclusion of all other diseases. A number of diseases affecting the musculo-skeletal system such as polymyalgia rheumatica, hypothyroidism, Parkinsonism may also produce symptoms resembling pain of bony origin.

The majority of painful episodes in osteoporosis are not due to the osteoporotic process itself but are associated with fractures, particularly vertebral fractures. Vertebral crush fractures result from a combination of the osteoporotic process and minor trauma. The extent of the fracture can vary from mild biconcave indentation of the vertebral body by the intervertebral disc to a complete anterior and posterior collapse, through various degrees of anterior wedging The most commonly affected vertebra are from T8 to L3 and, generally, the more severe the fracture, the more painful the episode. In a study, performed in 107 osteoporotic patients, divided into two groups according to the presence or absence of vertebral fractures, the assessment of bone pain by a visual analogue scale revealed that the majority and the severity of painful episodes were associated with the presence of vertebral fractures. Nevertheless, many vertebral fractures remain asymptomatic. Presenting pain is usually acute, diffuse, related to movement and often ameliorated by rest. The site of pain is often found to relate approximately to the anterior and posterior rami of the affected nerve roots. The pain is often of sufficient severity to be accompanied by shock and vomiting, and generally solves after two weeks of bed rest, but it may persist if a continuing pressure on surrounding structures is present or if the episode is repeated at another site.

Pain due to acute vertebral fracture can be extremely severe and therefore difficult to manage. In the initial management, the aim is to reduce the level of discomfort and improve mobility as soon as possible. Immobilization should be avoided, since prolonged immobilization is associated with bone loss. Alleviating pain and discomfort will generally improve mobility. Simple analgesics are sometimes sufficient to alleviate the pain, but in patients in whom simple analgesics do not provide adequate pain relief, non-steroidal anti-inflammatory drugs or narcotic analgesics may be necessary. To date a large number of clinical studies have shown calcitonin either by injection or by nasal spray to be effective in the acute stages of management of acute vertebral collapse. This treatment is able to determine a significant shortening of the painful phase in osteoporotic patients.

In addition to keeping the patient mobile, physiotherapy may help to strengthen the muscles of the back, leading to greater support of the spine and reducing the risk of future fractures. Some pain relief may also be achieved with the use of a transdermal electric nerve stimulation device (TENS).

Summary

Bone pain is a very common feature of many metabolic bone diseases such as metastatic bone disease, osteoporosis and Paget's disease of bone. The mechanism of pain is complex and depends on an increasing number of interrelated pathways and mediators. In general terms bone pain can be categorized as arising from one of the following mechanisms: a direct action on bone nociceptors or a secondary mechanical effect. There is little evidence that bone loss itself causes symptoms, until such time that a fracture occurs. Therefore, in osteoporosis, all the clinical manifestations are a direct or indirect consequence of fracture and thus, bone pain is the main clinical symptom. The most common causes of true bone pain, as opposed to joint pain, are trauma, osteoporosis and malignancy. Distinguishing among these different causes can be difficult and some diagnoses are often only made after exclusion of all other diseases. Pain due to acute vertebral fracture can be extremely severe and therefore difficult to manage. In the initial management, the aim is to reduce the level of discomfort and improve mobility as soon as possible. Immobilization should be avoided, since prolonged immobilization is associated with bone loss. Simple analgesics are sometimes sufficient to alleviate the pain, but in patients in whom simple analgesics do not provide adequate pain relief, non-steroidal anti-inflammatory drugs or narcotic analgesics may be necessary. To date a large number of clinical studies have shown calcitonin either by injection or by nasal spray to be effective in the acute stages of management of acute vertebral collapse. This treatment is able to determine a significant shortening of the painful phase in osteoporotic patients.

Suggested Reading

Gennari C, Agnusdei D. (1988) Calcitonin in bone pain management. *Curr Ther Res* 44: 712–722.

Gennari C, Agnusdei D, Camporeale A. (1991) Use of calcitonin in the treatment of bone pain associated with osteoporosis. *Calcif Tiss Int* 49: S9–13.

Pun KK, Chan LW. (1989) Analgesic effect of intranasal salmon calcitonin in the treatment of osteoporotic vertebral fractures. *Clin Ther* 11: 205–209.

14

Differential Diagnosis: Low Bone Mass

Michael Kleerekoper & Dorothy A. Nelson

Low bone mass is necessary but not sufficient for osteoporosis and fracture. It is the major contributor to the risk of fracture in an individual patient, but other factors also come into play. These include age, previous fracture, family history of fracture, and frequency of falls. Thus, when a patient has a bone mass measurement that results in a value that is lower than expected for age, and/or compared with young normals, it should be assumed that the risk of fracture is increased in this patient and intervention should be considered. Interventions can include pharmacologic therapy to stabilize or increase bone mass, lifestyle changes to protect the fragile skeleton, and physical activities that increase muscle strength and improve balance.

Age is a risk factor for osteoporosis over and above low bone mass. For every 5 years of age, risk increases by approximately 1.5. Some investigators have described two distinct types of osteoporosis depending on an individual's age and which bony component is most affected. Type I osteoporosis has been characterized by low bone mass in largely trabecular regions of the skeleton that is associated with the rapid bone loss of menopause. In this dichotomous model, type II osteoporosis affects mainly cortical bone and occurs later in the lifespan. Since trabecular bone has a greater surface area than cortical bone, it is more likely to be lost first and at a more rapid rate than cortical bone, no matter what the cause. Cortical bone is ultimately affected to a measurable and significant degree when bone loss proceeds unchecked. Thus, both compartments of bone are affected in osteoporosis and it is simpler and more accurate not to dichotomize the condition.

There is one cause of bone loss that appears to preferentially affect the cortical compartment, and that is hyperparathyroidism. Because of this phenomenon and the fact that differential diagnosis must take this possibility into account, it is helpful to measure bone mass at more than one skeletal site. However, this approach of multiple measurement sites can result in a conundrum when the results are discordant. If a mainly cortical site, such as the radial shaft, has low bone mineral content or density, and other sites such as the distal forearm, spine or hip are more normal, then hyperparathyroidism should be considered.

If there is discordance among sites, with at least one abnormally low, and hyperparathyroidism is not a likely cause, then it is probably best to err on the conservative side and assume that there is systemic low bone mass, or osteoporosis. There are only two possible explanations for obtaining different measurements at different sites : that the results really are different, or that they only appear to be different. In the first scenario, the sites may be different because of inherent differences in the bone(s) at the two sites. Alternatively, some factor may have affected the two sites differently during the patient's lifetime. Different measurement sites, even proximal and distal sites in the same long bone, do differ with respect to the proportion of cortical and cancellous bone. As discussed above, it is expected that skeletal sites with a larger proportion of cancellous bone will be affected the most by accelerated bone loss. Additionally, sites with more trabecular bone are presumed to be more metabolically active, but this too may depend on other factors such as proximity to fatty or hematopoietic marrow.

In the second scenario, where the discordance is more apparent than real, the explanation may be the error, although relatively small, that is inherent in bone mass measurements (1–2%). There are ranges of measurements, around the patient's measurement, that contain the "true" value. These ranges can be constructed using statistical tools that provide some level of confidence (such as 95%) that the true value falls within the range. If one site, by chance, is over or under estimated, and the other site is over or under estimated in the opposite direction (but still within the confidence interval), the results from the two sites may *appear* to be different. Thus, it is important to know and to keep in mind the level of error associated with bone mass measurements at the various sites, with various techniques, and at the clinician's own centre.

In summary, when bone mass measurements differ at two or more skeletal sites, it may be a reflection of differential rates of bone loss at the sites due to age or menopause, or it may suggest a secondary cause of bone loss that affects cortical more than cancellous bone. Alternatively, it may result from measurement error. In any case, a low bone mass at any skeletal site signals an increased fracture risk.

There are many epidemiologic data linking deficits in bone mass to increased fracture risk. Studies show that an abnormal measurement at any skeletal site is a good predictor of fracture risk. If the clinician wants to know about fracture risk at a specific site, such as the hip, then a measurement at that site is the best choice. In general, however, low bone mass is associated with increased fracture risk, and this relationship is stronger than that established for cholesterol levels and the risk of heart disease. This analogy, similar to that for high blood pressure and risk of stroke, is an important one because it emphasizes that abnormal measurements – high or low – are not in and of themselves disease. Rather, low bone mass like high serum cholesterol or blood pressure, signify a risk of some clinically significant event. And, as is the case for all of these abnormal measurements, they must be considered in the context of a clinical examination, the individual patient's history, and important personal characteristics such as age, body size, ethnicity, etc. In summary, low bone mass is perhaps the most important measurement in the diagnosis of osteoporosis and fracture risk, but a myriad of factors that affect bone mass and fracture risk must also be considered.

We must emphasize that low bone mass does not necessarily mean that bone has been lost since it is not possible to make such a dynamic statement on the basis of a single time point measurement. At any time the bone mass represents the difference between the peak bone mass attained during growth and the subsequent loss. This issue cannot be resolved unless serial bone mass data are available. However the lower the initial bone mass in seemingly healthy individuals, the more likely it is that bone loss has occurred. An important approach is not only to compare the individual's value to peak bone mass (T-score) but to an age, sex, and ethnicity adjusted reference interval (Z-score). With normal aging the T-score is low but the Z-score remains normal.

A value below the age, sex, and ethnicity adjusted reference interval should prompt a search for secondary causes of accelerated bone loss. i.e. a deficit in bone mass that cannot be fully accounted for by age or menopausal bone loss. The differential diagnosis of accelerated bone loss is extensive and includes

- hormone excess: parathyroid (primary or secondary)
                       thyroid (endogenous or exogenous)
                       cortisol (endogenous or exogenous)
- hormone deficiency: estrogen (premenopausal from any cause)
                       testosterone
                       vitamin D
- drugs: anticonvulsants
                       anticoagulants
                       antimetabolites
- diseases: malabsorption
                       systemic mastocytosis
                       paraplegia/tetraplegia
                       multiple myeloma

Summary

Low bone mass is an important clinical finding. It is the most precise method for assessing fracture risk in an individual subject, with risk prediction improved by additional data gathered from the history and physical examination. The pattern of low bone mass may provide clues to specific causes of accelerated bone loss such as hyperparathyroidism, where the value also plays an integral role in determining whether or not definitive treatment (parathyroidectomy or estrogen) is indicated. Finally, a very low value compared to individuals of the same age, sex, and ethnicity provides clues to important, often treatable, secondary causes of accelerated bone loss.

Suggested Reading

Cummings SR, Black DM, Nevitt MC et al. (1993) Bone density at various sites for prediction of hip fractures. *Lancet* 341: 72–75.

Gardsell P, Johnell O, Nilsson BE, Gullbert B. (1993) Predicting various fragility fractures in women by forearm bone densitometry: A follow-up study. *Calcif Tiss Int* 52: 348–353.

Greenspan SL, Maitland-Ramsey L, Myers E. (1996) Classification of osteoporosis in the elderly is dependent on site-specific analysis. *Calcif Tiss Int* 58: 409–414.

Hui SL, Slemenda CW, Johnston CC Jr. (1988) Age and bone mass as predictors of fracture in a prospective study. *J Clin Invest* 81: 1804–1809.

Kanis JA, Melton LJ III, Christiansen C et al. (1994) The diagnosis of osteoporosis. *J Bone Miner Res* 9: 1137–1141.

Kleerekoper M, Nelson D. (1988) Osteoporosis as a community health problem: Lessons learned from studying hypertension. *Henry Ford Hosp Med J* 36: 113–116.

Lafferty FW, Rowland DY. (1996) Correlations of dual-energy X-ray absorptiometry, quantitative computed tomography, and single photon absorptiometry with spinal and non-spinal fractures. *Osteoporosis Int* 6: 407–415.

Lai D, Rencken M, Drinkwater B et al. (1993) Site of bone density measurement may affect therapy decision. *Calcif Tiss Int* 53: 225–228.

Melton LJ III, Atkinson EJ, O'Fallon WM, Wahner HW. (1991) Long-term fracture risk prediction with bone mineral measurements made at various skeletal sites. *J Bone Miner Res* 6(S1): S136.

Miller PD, Bonnick SL, Rosen CJ. (1996) (for the Society for Clinical Densitometry). Clinical utility of bone mass measurements in adults: consensus of an international panel. *Sem Arth Rheum* 25: 361–372.

Nevitt MC, Cummings SR (1993) The Study of Osteoporotic Fractures Research Group. Type of fall and risk of hip and wrist fractures: the study of osteoporotic fractures. *J Am Geriatr Soc* 41: 1126–1234.

Ott SM. (1991) Methods of determining bone mass. *J Bone Miner Res* 6(2): S71–76.

Riggs BL, Melton LJ III (1983) Evidence for two distinct syndromes of involutional osteoporosis. *Am J Med* 75: 899.

Riis BJ, Christiansen C. (1988) Measurement of spinal or peripheral bone mass to estimate early postmenopausal bone loss? *Am J Med* 84: 646–653.

Ross PD, Davis JW, Epstein RS, Wasnich RD. (1991) Pre-existing fractures and bone mass predict vertebral fracture incidence in women. *Ann Intern Med* 114: 919–923.

WHO Study Group. (1994) Assessment of fracture risk and its application to screening for postmenopausal osteoporosis. *WHO Technical Report Series 843*. Geneva, Switzerland.

15

Differential Diagnosis: Falls

Jes B. Lauritzen & Klaus Hindso

Most osteoporosis-related fractures are a consequence of decreased bone density and falls.

Risk Factors for Falls

The risk factors for falls are numerous. In order to develop preventive strategies, it is necessary to identify risk factors associated with falls. According to a review by Myers et al, risk factors for falls can be categorized into the following nine groups (Table 15.1):

- general physical functioning
- gait, balance and physical performance
- musculoskeletal and neuromuscular measures
- demographic factors
- sensory impairments
- medical conditions
- indicators of general health
- medication us
- psychological, behavioral, social, and environmental factors.

However the relationship between level of physical activity and risk of falls is rather complex and a high activity level in the elderly may be accompanied with both increased and decreased risk of falls or fractures. Interventional studies to prevent falls have been performed and few studies targeting several potential risk factors have shown it possible to reduce the occurrence of falls.

Aging influences the postural control mechanisms, which include vision, vestibular function, proprioceptive and exteroceptive receptors, in addition to the central cerebral integration of these inputs. Muscle function also deteriorates with aging and the overall result may be a frail, elderly subject with unsteady, slow movements, tripping, swaying gait and an obvious need for aided support. Vitamin D3 and calcium supplementation in nursing home residents has been shown to reduce the rate of hip fractures, probably due to a reduction in the occurrence of falls, as BMD was unaltered, but unfortunately no information was available regarding muscle strength, balance and rate of falls. Nutritional factors

Table 15.1. Significant risk factors associated with falls.

---

1. General physical functioning

mobility
    ambulation/mobility   impaired stepping, stumbles
    trouble walking 400 m   walks with/without device
physical activity
    difficulty indoors   housebound
    >4 days spent in bed   days of limited activity
    goes shopping/visiting   > 10 activities past week
    large amount movement daily   frequency outdoors
    >2 different activities/week (protective)
    vigorous elderly:
            fell away from home
            fell on stairs
            more serious injury
disability
    physical disability   lower extremity disability
    specific activities of daily living
        ADL dependent, impaired
        difficulty:
                going up/down stairs   getting in/out bed
                dressing   bending down
                rising from chair
        can't rise from chair (protective) can't rise from chair
        nocturia 2–3 x/night

2. Gait, balance physical performance

poor tandem gait   gait, balance abnormalities
poor turning in place   > 12 steps to turn circle
turning reaching   poor one-foot stand
poor postural stress test   body sway
static/dynamic balance   abnormal push/pressure
                                    reaction
decreased Romberg   decreased standing on
                                    compliant surface

dizziness, vertigo, unsteady

3. Muscoloskeletal and neuromuscular measures

decreased muscle strength: handgrip, elbow, knee, hip
lower extremity peak torque/power   lower dorsiflexion power
muscle weakness/episodes   musculoskeletal problem
decreased ankle dorsiflexion   decreased ankle plantar
                                    flexion
plantar reflex abnormal   limited knee extension
peripheral neuropathy   abnormal position sense
decreased toe joint position sense   decreased sharp-dull
                                    discrimination
increased hand reaction time

Table 15.1. Continued.

4. Demographic	
age (protective)	age
female	Caucasian
5. Sensory	
vision problems	decreased visual acuity
impaired dark adaptation	double vision
errors in vertical perception	vertical perception problems
direct error in horizontal perception	direct visual error
cataracts	
6. Medical conditions	
number of medical conditions	heart disease
stroke	transient ischemic attack
Parkinson's disease	vertigo
dizziness	giddiness
faint / black out	neurotic disorder
depression	dementia
respiratory disorder	chronic lung disease
gastrointestinal disorder	incontinence: urinary or fecal
arthritis	osteoporosis
recent weight loss	hypotension
depression of pulse-pressure	systolic BP, heart rate
7. General health	
history of fall	history of injurious fall
self-reported decline in health	emotional problems
8. Medication use	
number of drugs	
drugs	
antidepressants	tranquilizer
non-phenothiazide tranquilizer	sedatives
hypnotics	psychotropic drugs
psychoactive drugs	antipsychotics
vasodilators	NSAID
diuretics	cardiac medications (protective)
cardiac medications	antihypertensive
oral hypoglycemics	adverse drug reaction
9. Psychological, behavorial, social and environmental factors	
behavorial factors	
lower safety preference	no fear of falling
physical restraints needed	
psychological/mental/cognitive impairment	
confusion after hospitalization	
reversible condition affecting cognition	

Table 15.1. Continued.

social/physical environment	
living alone	social interactions (less)
social activities (low)	environmental hazards
household type	

may be important, but difficult to quantitate, but malnutrition and undernourishment may be associated with other known risk factors for falls. Excessive alcohol intake increases the risk of falls.

No general test for fall risk estimation is available, but postural sway test, Romberg test, measuring ortostatic hypotension, or muscle strength tests may give some valuable information. Tinetti et al. have proposed an index for chronic fallers. A recent prospective study from the Lyon-group performed fall-risk status measurements (gait speed, tandem walk score, calf circumference, and visual acuity) in addition to femoral BMD and calcaneal broadband ultrasonic attenuation (BUA), and they found a relation to subsequent risk of hip fracture. Femoral BMD and calcaneal BUA and fall-risk score had approximately the same predictive ability.

Occurrence of Falls

The annual rate of falls is 28–35% among home dwellers more than 65 years of age and 3242 % of subjects older than 75 years of age sustain at least one fall a year. For nursing home residents the occurrence is 1.5 falls per resident per year, and the annual rate of fallers is higher than 80%. Repeat fallers in nursing homes account for more than 40% of all falls among the residents.

Most falls do not cause major injuries, but the risk of injuries following falls in the elderly is very high. The incidence of falls leading to medical treatment in the elderly is 6–19 per 1000 persons per year. More than 10% of elderly people more than 90 years of age will be treated in hospital due to a fall within one year. In a Danish nursing home the proportion of falls on the hip compared with all falls was 24% in women and 13% in men and the incidence of falls on the hip was 36 per 100 residents per year in women and 16 in male residents. In case of impact to the hip the risk of hip fracture in women was 0.25 and 0.33 in men.

The following conditions are of importance for a fall to cause a hip fracture: impact near the hip; protective reflexes; local soft tissue energy absorption; and bone strength. Preventive measures against hip fractures should be aimed at these various fundamental risk factors. More than 90% of hip fractures are related to a direct impact to the hip, although only one fourth of impacts to the hip in the elderly lead to a hip fracture. Rarely a hip fracture occurs without a direct trauma. In falls on the hip compared to other falls the odds ratio for a hip fracture is 17.1–21.7.

Force and Energy in Falls on the Hip

In unprotected falls performed by stuntmen on a force platform the effective load acting on the hip was 35 per cent of the body weight. The force obtained in these falls on the hip showed a peak force of 3.5 kN (energy 113 Joules) in a female weighing 60 kg.

Protective Responses

The initial potential energy in falls can be reduced significantly by protective responses as shown by stuntmen. Elderly people experience minor and other traumas compared to young subjects. Reduced reaction time and slow coordination has been found related to risk of fractures. Many patients with hip fractures are admitted from nursing homes, and this group is characterized by disturbances in their neuromuscular functions.

Energy Absorption

Energy absorption in soft tissue can be a more important factor than bone strength in relation to hip fractures. Experimental studies have shown that the energy absorption may account for up to 75% of the energy, and partially explain why overweight protects against hip fractures.

Women with hip fractures weigh on average 5 kg less compared with controls. In addition women with hip fractures seem to have less soft tissue covering their hips compared with controls even when adjusted for body mass index.

About 42% of all falls sustained within home occur in the bathroom. Impact attenuation of floor coverings may have a minor effect on the peak force in case of falls even when one compares tiles with a carpet floor covering.

Bone Strength

The fracture threshold in the hip has been studied in cadavers and the breaking strength ranges from 5.5–9.2 kN in young people ($n = 9$) and the breaking strength in the hip ranges from 2.0–6.3 kN in old subjects ($n = 8$). The impact site and the body mass index are strong predictors of hip fracture risk.

The type of impacts leading to either a femoral neck or a trochanteric fracture is still unsolved. A lateral impact may be more likely to lead to a neck fracture, while a posterior/lateral impact may lead to more trochanteric hip fractures. The various types of falls in the elderly has not yet been fully investigated.

Risk of Hip Fracture

Numerous risk factors for hip fracture exist, and preventive actions must focus on several modalities in order to prevent hip fractures. Residents in nursing homes, elderly patients admitted to hospitals for dizziness, falls, fractures and compromised mobility are certainly at risk. Home dwellers as such with the above mentioned risk factors are also a target group for protectors.

Analyses have shown that use of hip protectors are indeed cost-saving, due to the high cost of hip fracture treatment and rehabilitation and the substantial and immediate protective effect from the hip protectors.

All elderly women and men with increased risk of falls and osteoporosis should be considered candidates for hip protectors, besides other preventive measures.

Conclusion

The risk of falls is multifactorial, and the prevention must adapt to this fact. The cascade of events leading to fracture involves: a fall, protective responses, energy absorption and bone strength. Prevention of falls and fractures must be multifactorial due to the many risk factors related to the elements provoking falls and the subsequent cascade of events leading to fracture (Table 15.2). The target groups are frail elderly subjects, who are institutionalized/hospitalized or home dwellers.

Table 15.2. Preventive actions against falls.

• Maintaining physical activity. Balance exercises. Endurance exercises.
• Adjustments and avoiding fall hazards in the home environment
• Securing a qualitative and quantitative diet
• Adjustment of medication interfering with neuromuscular status
• Supplementation of vitamin D3 and calcium among nursing home residents
• Use of external hip protectors

Summary

A fall and a trauma are almost obligatory events for a fracture to occur, except for osteoporosis related spine fractures, where spontaneous fractures are more common, at least the specific trauma may be difficult to define. Most falls do not cause major injuries, but the risk of fractures in falls among elderly is very high due to pre-existing silent osteoporosis. As a consequence, the type of fall is the main predominator of the type of osteoporosis fracture the elderly subject will sustain. The force acting on the hip in falls from standing height is about 3.5 kN, and while the breaking strength of the hip in the elderly ranges from about 2–6 kN a hip fracture will only occur in susceptible subjects in case of unprotected falls of the hip.

The risk factors for falls are numerous, and those elderly experiencing repeated falls tend to have more functional disability, impaired mobility, neuromuscular and vestibular dysfunction, in addition to poor vision. Aging interferes with sensory and postural modalities and increases the risk of falls. CNS-active drugs and alcohol are also important risk factors. The occurrence of falls is high among nursing home residents and frail elderly community dwellers.

Preventing falls is difficult, however non-pharmacological multifactorial intervention programs have shown 9–12% fewer falls corresponding to an odds ratio between 0.74 and 0.85.

Vitamin D3 and calcium supplementation in nursing home residents have been shown to reduce the rate of fractures by one third, probably due to a reduction in the rate of falls.

Efficient hip protective systems have been developed and may be a significant factor in the prevention of hip fractures, and clinical studies have shown a 50–80% reduction in the rate of hip fractures. More than 90% of all hip fractures can theoretically be prevented by hip protectors and those who may benefit most are frail elderly home dwellers, nursing home residents and elderly patients admitted to hospitals.

A multifactorial intervention to reduce the occurrence of falls and consequently fractures is mandatory.

Suggested Reading

Dargent-Molina P, Haushesse E, Hans D, Favier F, Grandjean H, Baudoin C, Schott AM, Bréart G, Meunier PJ. (1996) Fall related factors and risk of hip fracture: the EPIDOS prospective study.*Lancet* 348: 145–149.

Greenspan SL, Resnick NM, Maitland LA, Lipsitz LA, Myers ER, Hayes WC. (1994) Fall severity and bone mineral density as risk factors for hip fracture in ambulatory elderly *JAMA* 271: 128–33.

Hayes WC, Myers ER, Robinovitch SN, van den Kronenburg A, Courtney AC, McMahon TA (1996) Etiology and prevention of age-related hip fractures. *Bone* 18: 77S-86S.

Jäntti P. (1993) Falls in the elderly. With special reference to testing posture control and risk factors. *Acta Universitatis Tamperensis* Ser A 362. University of Tampere.

Lauritzen JB. (1997) Hip fractures. Epidemiology, risk factors, falls, energy absorption, hip protectors, and prevention. *Dan Med Bull* 44: 155–168.

Lauritzen JB, Hindso K. (1997) Prevention of hip fractures with hip protectors. *Orthopaedics Int Edn* 5: 125–130.

Lauritzen JB, Petersen MM, Lund B. (1993) Effect of external hip protectors on hip fractures. *Lancet* 341: 11–3.

Myers AH, Young Y, Langlois JA. (1996) Prevention of falls in the elderly *Bone* 18: 87S-101S.

Tinetti ME, Williams TF, Mayewski R. (1986) Fall risk index for elderly patients based on number of chronic disabilities *Am J Med* 80: 429–434.

Tinetti ME, Baker DI, McAvay GA. (1994) A multifactorial intervention to reduce the risk of falling among elderly living in the community. *N Engl J Med* 331: 821–827.

16

Prevention During Growth and Young Adulthood

Charles W. Slemenda

There is little question that the response of the skeleton to stimuli such as dietary factors and exercise is greatest during periods of rapid growth. Although the precise timing of peak bone mass differs somewhat among the various skeletal sites, by age 18 the skeleton is nearly fully developed and only very modest increases in bone mass or density can be expected after the cessation of longitudinal growth.

Calcium

Randomized intervention studies aimed at increasing peak bone mass have been limited to calcium clinical trials. At least four such trials have been completed, and all have shown modest (+2–5%) short-term gains in bone mineral content and density associated with 300–1000 mg/day supplements. The gains in bone density do not appear to be larger in those clinical trials with larger calcium doses, and only one study has shown a consistently larger effect in those children who entered the trial with lower dietary calcium intake. Calcium balance studies have suggested that children and adolescents may continue to increase net calcium absorption up to about 1500 mg/day, although precise estimates of the maximum useful calcium dose are not available.

The issue of whether or not these benefits of calcium intake can be maintained upon cessation of supplementation remains to be completely resolved. Three of the four published studies have reported slower post-supplement bone gain in previously supplemented children compared with control group subjects, resulting in a loss of the calcium benefit within 2–3 years post-supplementation. The most recent study has raised the possibility, however, that maintenance of this beneficial effect may be possible, although longer follow-up of the study subjects will be required. Increased calcium intake, whether from dietary or other sources, is unlikely to provide long-term benefits unless these higher levels of calcium intake are maintained for long periods. Observational studies in older adults are consistent in this regard, demonstrating 3–6% higher bone densities in those women with high calcium intakes in childhood and adolescence.

It is often recognized that some populations, particularly those in developing nations, have habitually low calcium intakes, and yet rarely suffer osteoporotic fractures. This difference in fracture rates, however, probably reflects the high levels of physical activity and greater strength that is common among the elderly members of these societies. In fact, the few studies that have actually examined bone density in low calcium intake areas of Africa have found density to be lower than in comparable European populations. Thus, the international data are consistent in this regard as well.

It has been suggested that other dietary components, particularly phosphoric acid from carbonated beverages, caffeine, protein and sodium, may negatively influence calcium balance. Few studies, aside from short-term laboratory experiments, have addressed these issues in free-living subjects, and none has been studied in clinical trials. There are already many reasons to believe that lower sodium, caffeine and protein intakes may be beneficial, but the effects of changes in these patterns on peak bone density remain to be established.

Physical Activity - Potential Benefits

Clinical trials to rigorously determine the magnitude of exercise effects on the growing skeleton have not been done. Studies of self-selected athletes raise the possibility of selection bias, which might favor the entry of those with greater muscle mass and bone density into studies. This bias is impossible to avoid in observational studies. The observational data, however, are consistent regarding the types of activities needed to influence skeletal density, assuming that biases do not play an important role in what has been reported. Weight-bearing activities, particularly those that involve impact loading, such as gymnastics, basketball, volleyball, figure skating, and similar endeavors, yield more favorable skeletal effects than swimming or cycling, both of which provide minimal skeletal loading. The potential magnitude of exercise effects appears to be greater than that of calcium supplementation, although direct comparisons are not possible. Children in the uppermost quarter of physical activity, using either self- or parent-reported data, had, in one study, 8–12% higher bone densities than children in the lowest 25% of activity, and gained significantly more bone over time than did low activity children.

Recently published data on young girls involved in gymnastics or figure skating provide further evidence regarding the importance of high impact activities. Several studies of these groups have shown that, even in the presence of high frequencies of menstrual disturbances (oligo- and amenorrhea), these girls have higher average bone densities than normal controls. And, unlike many other sports, these activities favor smaller, lighter children who are unlikely to be selected for large skeletons. Both of these sports involve repetitive, high impact activities, and both involve equipment (i.e., skates, gymnastics apparatus) which help increase the speed and forces to levels beyond those seen in other sports. Before specific activities can be recommended, however, studies into the effects of these activities on other musculoskeletal components (e.g., the joints) should be completed.

Physical Activity - Potential Risks

Extremely intense physical activity can be accompanied by amenorrhea in young women. Although there are exceptions, as noted above, this condition is usually associated with reduced bone density. The balance between adequate and excessive activity is not difficult to achieve, although it may be difficult to convince some athletes to reduce the intensity of their activities. Few data exist to evaluate the interaction between diet and activity, but increased caloric intake may be useful in the prevention or resolution of activity induced amenorrhea, although there have not been convincing clinical studies to support this concept. It is less well appreciated that young men with extremely high activity levels may also have low bone mass. Runners, for example, have been shown to have 5–15% lower bone densities than control subjects, although it has been argued that this is primarily due to lower body weights. Ultimately, however, athletic activity that results in disturbances of normal gonadal function or disturbed eating patterns requires intervention.

Anorexia Nervosa

A discussion of factors influencing peak bone mass and ultimate fracture risk would be incomplete without consideration of this devastating condition. Young women who develop anorexia may have severe osteopenia or osteoporosis at the time of diagnosis. Treatment of the underlying psychological problem and recovery of the weight lost are associated with higher bone densities in women followed over a decade or more. However, even among those women with the most complete recoveries there may remain a skeletal density deficit. In those with poor recoveries this deficit may be as large as 1–2 standard deviations at the time of peak bone mass resulting in a substantial increase in fracture risk. Specific treatments for these skeletal problems have not been developed for young women. Treatment of the frequently accompanying amenorrhea with estrogens has not been shown to correct the deficits in skeletal mass, and other therapies currently available for older women have not been tested in children or adolescents.

Suggested Reading

Bonjour J-P. (1997) Calcium-enriched foods and bone mass growth. *J Clin Invest* 99(6):1287–1294.

Crosby LO, Kaplan FS, Pertschuk MJ et al. (1985) The effect of anorexia nervosa on bone morphometry in young women. *Clin Orthop* 201:271–277.

Drinkwater BL, Breumner B and Chestnut C. (1990) Menstrual history as a determinant of current bone density in athletes. *JAMA* 263:545–548.

Johnston CC, Miller JZ, Slemenda C et al. (1992) Calcium supplementation and increases in bone mineral density in children. *N Engl J Med* 327:82–87.

Lloyd T, Andon MB, Rollings N et al. (1993) Calcium supplementation and bone mineral density in adolescent girls. *JAMA* 270:841–844.

Robinson TL, Snow-Harter C, Taaffe DR et al. (1995) Gymnasts exhibit higher bone mass than runners despite similar prevalence of amenorrhea and oligomenorrhea. *J Bone Miner Res* 10:26–35.

Theintz G, Buchs B, Rizzoli et al. (1992) Longitudinal monitoring of bone mass accumulation in healthy adolescents: evidence for a marked reduction after 16 years of age at the levels of lumbar spine and femoral neck in female subjects. *J Clin Endocrinol Metab* 75:1060–1065.

Slemenda C, Johnston CC. (1993) High intensity activities in young women: site specific effects among figure skaters. *Bone Miner* 20:125–132.

Slemenda C, Reister TK, Hui SL et al. (1994) Influences on skeletal mineralization in children and adolescents: evidence for varying effects of sexual maturation and physical activity. *J Pediatr* 125:201–207.

17

Prevention Early After Menopause: Hormonal

Nikolai A. Manassiev & John Stevenson

The menopause signals a major transition in female physiology. During the reproduction years, a woman's ovaries mainly produce estradiol, with levels in the blood varying between 180 and 1500 pmol/l depending on the day of the cycle. Following the menopause, estradiol levels are commonly below 110 pmol/l. Since estradiol is a hormone which affects many biological processes, its decline starts a chain of events which lead to the development of vasomotor symptoms, genitourinary atrophy, osteoporosis and cardiovascular disease.

The Effect of Estrogen on Bone

The development of osteoporosis depends both on the peak bone mass attained and its subsequent loss. Peak bone mass is achieved in early adulthood and is largely genetically determined. This has been confirmed in studies comparing bone mass in twins and in studies of racial groups that have migrated. To a lesser extend, bone mass is dependent on diet, exercise, alcohol consumption, smoking, drugs (e.g. corticosteroids, contraceptive pills, liver enzyme inducers), parity and the presence or absence of estrogens. The rate of change in bone mass depends on the way various factors affect the bone mass through altering the balance between bone resorption and formation. Estrogens seem to have a central role in regulating bone mass.

The development of osteoporosis results from an imbalance between bone resorption and bone formation. The loss of gonadal function and aging are the two most important factors. Starting around the fourth or fifth decade of life, men and women lose 0.3 –0.5% of bone a year. After the loss of the gonadal function, this is increased by up to tenfold in women due to an increase in bone turnover.

Mechanism of Action

Estrogens are thought to affect the bone both directly and indirectly.

Direct Actions

Studies on osteoblast-like osteosarcoma cells and in human osteoblast-like cells have shown that these possess estrogen receptors. Estrogen binds to the receptors and, through the classical estrogen receptor medicated mechanism, leads to response from the cells which may include the production of type I collagen and transforming growth factor-beta (TGF- β).

Estrogen also acts through locally produced factors: cytokines, growth factors and prostaglandins. Cytokines (IL-1, IL-6), tumor necrosis factors and TGF-β, are potent inducers of bone resorption and osteoclast formation. They are secreted by stromal cells in the bone marrow and by osteoclasts. It has been suggested that estrogens are potent inhibitors of IL-6 and perhaps of other cytokines. The changes in bone turnover are most pronounced where metabolic activity is high such as in trabecular bone.

Indirect Actions

Estrogens may alter the set point at which the parathyroid hormone (PTH) responds to calcium, thus reducing the PTH secretion and the rate of bone turnover. It may also stimulate intestinal calcium absorption by enhancing renal $1,25(OH)_2D_3$ synthesis. It may also enhance secretion of calcitonin, a hormone which inhibits bone resorption.

The Case for Early or Late Intervention with Estrogen

The decreased bone mass seen following the menopause and the development of osteoporosis represent a major public health issue. Osteoporosis and fractures occur much more often in women than in men. One standard deviation decrease in bone density leads to a threefold increase of the risk of fracture. For women aged 50, the lifetime risk of osteoporotic fracture is 30–40%, more than three time that in men.

Several factors are considered to play a role:

(1) women have a lower skeletal mass at maturity;

(2) because of the menopause, the bone loss is greater in women than in men;

(3) life expectancy is greater for women;

(4) women seem to suffer falls more frequently than men.

Public awareness about osteoporosis is increasing and more and more women require information from their health providers about fracture risk and osteoporosis prevention and treatment. Currently estrogens are one of the most potent medications for preventing bone loss and increasing bone mass after it has been lost following the menopause.

There is no definition in the literature what is early and late postmenopause. If we consider that many women spend about 30 years in menopause (between the ages of 50 and 80), then the first 10 years or so postmenopause may be considered early, and thereafter the late postmenopause. The menopause indicates a significant reduction in ovarian estrogen production and thus a time when sex hormones can start to be replaced. There is evidence that, in the early years following surgical or natural menopause, there is a period of accelerated bone loss, which in later life decreases but still continues into old age. During these early years, the bone microstructure may be adversely compromised with perforation and loss of trabecular elements. The process of architectural damage is probably irreversible, even if estrogens are given later in life. Early intervention will maximize the number and integrity of trabecular structures remaining in the bone tissue and will help to retain bone strength. When estrogens are given late in the menopause the increase in bone density is only due to the increased mass/thickness of the remaining trabecular elements. Thus the bone may never regain its original strength. Nevertheless estrogens can benefit bone strength and reduce fracture risk even in women with established osteoporosis by the conservation and strengthening of these remaining trabecular elements. Thus late intervention may still give considerable benefit in term of fracture risk reduction.

The menopause is also associated with vasomotor symptoms, insomnia, urogenital atrophy and psychological and psychosomatic symptoms in the vast majority of women. Hormone replacement treatment (HRT) will effectively treat these symptoms. In addition, if HRT is given earlier in the menopause, its side effects (withdrawal bleeds, premenstrual syndrome-like symptoms, nausea, headache, bloatedness, muscle cramps) may be more easily accepted by women. The main disadvantage of early intervention with HRT is the necessity of prolonged treatment which requires long term compliance, and the potential increase in the risk of any long-term adverse effects. The benefits of prolonged HRT on lipids and lipoproteins include reduction of the incidence of CVD and stroke, preventing unfavorable changes in lipids, glucose and insulin metabolism, coagulation and fibrinolysis which are seen following the menopause. HRT also improves muscle strength, increases skin thickness and may prevent the development of Alzheimer's diseases. Furthermore, since prevention is better than cure, there are compelling reasons to start estrogen replacement as soon as estrogen deficiency occurs.

Evidence of Hormone Replacement Therapy Efficacy on the Skeleton

In many older studies, the site of measurement is the wrist or the metacarpal bones. This may not truly correlate with the bone density in the spine and the hip. Often, there is no distinction between surgical-induced and natural menopause. Following early surgical menopause, the rate of bone loss may be greater than seen with natural menopause. The method of measurement and its coefficient of variation is important. For some methods, precision is 1–2.5% which is well within the expected yearly bone loss or gain, thus longer follow-up studies are required.

The presentation of results is not always clear. For example, expressing group data as means and standard errors conceals the fact that some 8–15% do not conserve bone with standard therapy.

Treatment Regimens

Estrogens with or without Progestogens: Oral Treatments

There are two main oral estrogens: conjugated equine estrogens (CEE) and 17-β estradiol (E_2). Oestrone sulphate is also available but is used to much lesser extent. CEEs are available in two dosages: 0.625 mg and 1.25 mg. They consist mainly of estrone (50%) and equilin (25%) but virtually no estradiol. 17-β estradiol is available in 1, 2 and 4 mg tablets. Taken by mouth, it is transformed mainly to estrone. All orally available estrogens undergo first pass hepatic metabolism and are transformed to estrone and estriol. This produces favorable effects on lipids and lipoproteins, increasing HDL and decreasing LDL, but may increase the renin-substrate and certain haemostatic factors. Synthetic 17-α-alkylated estrogens, such as ethinyl estradiol, are not used in HRT because they are not oxidized by 17-β estradiol dehydrogenase and therefore have a greater effect on the liver.

The bone conserving dose of oral estrogens is 0.625 mg for CEE, 1 to 2 mg E_2 or 1.5 mg for estrone. Unopposed estrogen is used in hysterectomized women whilst progestogen addition for 12–14 days each month is necessary in non-hysterectomized women to prevent endometrial hyperplasia and carcinoma. Different progestogens in equipotent dosages will be equally effective in preventing endometrial disease, but will have different metabolic effects. More androgenic progestogens, such as 19-nortestosterone derivatives in dosages of 1 mg norethisterone acetate (NETA) or 75 μg levonorgestrel, will provide a very good cycle control. NETA may also have additional bone sparing effects of its own.

Less androgenic progestogens, such as C-21 pregnane derivatives medroxyprogesterone and dydrogesterone, have fewer side effects such as acne, greasy skin and fluid retention.

In order to avoid monthly withdrawal bleeds, estrogens and progestogens may be given continuously as continuous combined HRT. After 6 months of such treatment, some 60–70% of truly postmenopausal women will be amenorrhoeic, which may greatly increase their compliance. However, continuous combined HRT has been less well studied with regard to its metabolic effects.

Parenteral Estrogens

Parenteral estrogens can be administered in the form of patches, implants or gels. In the case of patches and gels, estrogen in the form of estradiol is delivered through the skin, whilst implants are inserted subcutaneously, where they slowly release estradiol. In this way, the first-pass metabolism in the liver is avoided and much smaller amounts are needed. Patches are changed once or twice weekly, and implants are usually inserted every 6 months, which may improve compliance. The patches deliver estradiol at a steady rate, and this way peaks and troughs are avoided. The implants have a high initial peak which may last up to 2–4 weeks. Once inserted, they cannot be easily removed, and estrogen levels may build up with frequent use. It is therefore necessary to monitor estrogen levels before a new implant is inserted and to delay administration until the levels fall to under 500 pmol/l.

The estradiol gel (estrogel) contains 1.5 mg estradiol in 2.5 g of gel (two measures of 1.25 g each), which delivers approximately 75 µg of estradiol through the skin. The suggested initial dosage is one or two applications of 2.5 g of gel daily (two to four measures).

Bone sparing doses are 50 µg/day for the patches, 50 mg for the implants and 2.5 g daily for estradiol gel (1.5 mg estradiol).

Table 17.1. Bone-conserving doses of estrogens. High-dose is the dose suggested for use in young women with premature menopause whereas low-dose is the dose suggested for use in elderly women. Bone density monitoring may be necessary in such cases.

Estrogen	Normal	High-dose	Low-dose
Conjugated equine estrogens	0.625 mg	1.25 mg	0.3 mg*
Estrone sulphate	1.5 mg	3 mg	0.75 mg*
Oral estradiol 17	2 mg	4 mg	1 mg
Transdermal estradiol 17(patch)	0.05 mg	0.1 mg	0.025 mg
Subcutaneous estradiol 17	50 mg	100 mg	25 mg

*achieved by giving 1 tablet on alternate days.

Norethisterone

Estrogens are contra-indicated in some women, especially those with estrogen-dependent tumors, such as breast cancer or uterine cancer, or with thromboembolic phenomena. In those patients, progestogens as sole treatment may provide symptomatic relief and will prevent bone loss. Norethisterone, 5 mg bd continuously, will increase the bone density in early postmenopausal women, followed for up to 3 years. The mechanism of action is not clear, but its androgenic properties may play a role. Less androgenic progestogens such as medroxyprogesterone acetate have no effect on bone density.

Tibolone

Tibolone is a synthetic compound with weak hormonal properties. Comparative animal studies have demonstrated that the estrogenic properties of tibolone are one fiftieth of those of ethinylestradiol, its progestogenic properties one eighth of those of norethisterone, and its androgenic properties one third of those of norethisterone. It effectively relieves vasomotor symptoms and does not stimulate the endometrium. The standard dose of 2.5 mg/day leads to an increase in bone density in the forearm and the lumbar spine. Around 6% non-responders to treatment were found after 2 years.

Testosterone

Testosterone is produced in small amounts in women. Some 50–60% of testosterone originate from the ovary whilst the rest is produced by peripheral conversion of adrenal androstenedione and androstenedione sulphate. Overall, the ovary contributes about two-thirds and the adrenal about one-third of the circulating testosterone. Testosterone is largely protein bound and only the free fraction is active. Testosterone has anabolic and androgenic effects. It increases muscle bulk, increases bone density and stimulates peripheral hair growth and sebaceous gland secretion. Oral testosterone esters have adverse metabolic effects. Testosterone can be administered non-orally to women by implants.

Nandrolone decanoate, 50 mg i.m., administered every 3 to 4 weeks, leads to significant increase of bone density when used in both early postmenopausal women and in women with established osteoporosis. Gains in bone density in the femoral neck and the lumbar spine are observed. The side effects most often encountered are raised blood pressure, leg oedema, voice hoarseness and facial hair, which are seen in up to 50% of the women receiving nandrolone.

Adverse Effects and Risks of Postmenopausal Hormone Replacement Therapy

Withdrawal bleeding is one of the reasons why the majority of women starting HRT stop after a short time. With sequential HRT most women will experience regular withdrawal bleeds. The duration is between 3 and 7 days and the periods are generally lighter than in reproductive years. If the bleeding starts on or after the eleventh day of the progestogen phase, this usually means that the endometrium has undergone an adequate secretory transformation. If women do not bleed on sequential HRT or on continuous combined HRT, this indicates that the endometrium is atrophic and does not need investigation.

The lifetime risk of endometrial cancer is about 3% for women aged 50. Unopposed estrogen increases this risk 4–6 times after 5 years of use and 10 times after 10 years of use. The addition of progestogens for at least 12 days each month will reduce the risk of developing endometrial cancer virtually to the background rate. Endometrial assessment is only required in women on sequential therapy whose withdrawal bleed changes in amount, timing or duration. Women on continuous combined or sequential HRT who were amenorrhoeic but started to bleed after a period of time will also need to be investigated.

Breast cancer is a major cause of cancer death in women in UK. The lifetime risk for a woman aged 50 and living in the UK is about 8–10%. The fear that HRT administered to postmenopausal women will increase the breast cancer risk is one of the major reasons why many women will not take HRT in the menopause and many doctors will advise against it. However, evidence that HRT increases breast cancer risk is not conclusive, and there is evidence of a lower mortality rate in women on HRT who develop breast cancer.

Until very recently, HRT was not thought to be associated with an increased risk of venous thromboembolism. Some recent case controlled studies have suggested a two- to fourfold increase of venous thromboembolism in HRT users compared to age-matched non-users. However, there are concerns about these studies. Nevertheless, women with previous venous thromboembolic events suggestive of thrombophilia or with a strong family history of thromboembolic disorders may warrant haemostatic investigation prior to treatment. There are reasons for recommending the use of transdermal HRT in such women.

Summary

Hormonal prevention of osteoporosis with estrogens is a major advance in preventive medicine. Such treatment leads to improved longevity and quality of life. It also produces relief of menopausal symptoms and decreases the incidence of other menopause related conditions affecting the urogenital, cardiovascular and central nervous systems. It may, however, have some undesirable adverse effects. They may be minor, as in the case of abdominal bloatedness, muscle cramps, headache, breast tenderness, or unscheduled vaginal bleeding. They may be also major, as in the case of the unresolved questions about the long-term safety of estrogen on the breast. Careful selection of patients and careful monitoring of therapy will help keep the adverse effects and risks to a minimum. Early intervention with hormone replacement is clearly an important strategy for the prevention of postmenopausal osteoporosis.

Suggested Reading

Abdalla HI, Hart DM, Lindsay R et al. (1985) Prevention of bone mineral loss in postmenopausal women by norethisterone. *Obstet Gynecol* 66: 789–92.

Cristiansen C, Cristiansen MS, Larsen NE, Transbol I. (1982) Pathophisiological mecanisms of estrogen effect on bone metabolism. Dose-response relationships in early postmenopausal women. *J Clin Endocrinol Metab* 55: 1124–30.

Ettinger B, Genant HK, Steiger P, Madvig P. (1992) Low-dosage micronized 17ß-estrodiol prevents bone loss in postmenopausal women. *Am J Obstet Gynecol* 166: 479–88.

Gutthan SP, Rodriguez LAG, Castellsague J, Oliart AD. (1997) Hormone replacement therapy and risk of venous thromboembolism: population based case-control study *BMJ* 314: 796–800.

Harris ST, Genant HK, Baylink DJ et al. (1991) The effects of estrone (Ogen) on spinal bone density of postmenopausal women. *Arch Intern Med* 151: 1980–84.

Lindsay R, Hart DM, Forrest C, Baird C. (1980) Prevention of spinal osteoprosis in oophorectomised women. *Lancet* ii: 1151–54.

Manolagos SC, Jilka RL. (1995) Bone marrow, cytokines, and bone remodeling. *N Engl J Med* 332: 305–11.

Marsden J, Sacks NPM. (1996) Hormone replacement therapy and breast cancer. *Endocrine-related Cancer* 3: 81–97.

Prelevic GM, Bartram C, Wood J et al. (1996) Comparative effects on bone mineral density of tibolone, transdermal estrogen and oral estrogen-progestogen therapy in postmenopausal women. *Gynecol Endocrinol* 10: 413–420.

Stevenson JC. (1996) Benefits and risks of hormone therapy. In: Weatherall DJ, Ledingham JGG, Warren DA (eds) *Oxford Textbook of Medicine,* 3rd edn. Oxford University Press, Oxford pp. 1813–15.

Stevenson JC, Cust MP, Gangar KF et al. (1990) Effects of trandermal versus oral hormonal replacement therapy on bone density in spine and proximal femur in postmenopausal women. *Lancet* 336: 265–9.

Studd J, Savvas M, Waston N et al. (1990) The relationship between plasma estradiol and the increase in bone density in postmenopausal women after treatment with subcutaneous hormone implants. *Am J Obstet Gynecol* 163: 1474–9.

18

Prevention Early After Menopause: Non-hormonal Intervention

Aurelio Rapado

Prevention should be directed towards the optimization of peak bone mass. Unfortunately major contributors (race and heredity) are unchangeable and the impact of other potential factors such as exercise and nutrition is of uncertain value.

Nevertheless as non-hormonal factors account for the large inter-regional differences in the incidence of osteoporosis, lifestyle factors are of great importance in determining bone mass. In this setting, avoiding risk factors from adolescence could play a role in preventing fractures later in life

There are some key indications to start bone loss prevention early after menopause. These include the presence of strong risk factors as premature menopause, prolonged secondary amenorrhea, primary hypogonadism. Other conditions include a previous fragility fracture, radiographic evidence of vertebral deformity, significant loss of height or thoracic kyphosis. Low body weight is also a risk factor as this is related to the postmenopausal production of estrogen and to a decreased weight on the skeleton. In fact there is evidence that loss of mineral in the forearm is reduced in women who are heavier.

Different nutritional factors have been associated with an increased risk of osteoporosis and these could be controlled at this stage. Calcium and vitamin D recommended daily allowances are amply covered in nowadays, but sunshine exposition could contribute to a better absorption and metabolism. Avoiding excessive amounts of meat and fish will reduce the rate of sulphate elimination, hence inducing urinary calcium loss and a negative calcium balance. Caffeine-containing drinks can increase the urinary excretion rate of calcium but its contribution to osteoporosis is at best circumstantial. High sodium diet increases the urinary excretion of calcium due to a decrease in renal tubular reabsorption which might stimulate the secretion of parathormone and thus increase the activation frequency of bone.

Smoking affects skeletal mass loss and fracture risk in several ways and the skeletal protection provided by estrogen replacement therapy is lost in those who smoke.

Alcohol use alters calcium regulating hormones, reduces bone formation and results in osteopenia. Heavy alcohol consumption increases hip fracture risk.

Certain drugs such as corticosteroids, thyroxin, heparin, lithium, cytotoxic chemotherapy of anticonvulsivants, increase bone loss and reduce bone formation through their effect on mineral metabolism and bone cell functions. Due to considerable variation between individual patients in their resistance to osteopenic effect it is mandatory to monitor the dose and keep it to a minimum.

The tropic effect of physical activity on the skeleton has stimulated the use of many exercise regimens to prevent bone loss. Weight-bearing exercises are the most effective but the threshold, type, degree and periodicity that are optimal for bone mass is not known. For various reasons the impact of exercise regimens, particularly strength and aerobic, is small and does not prevent bone loss due to estrogen deficiency. Weightbearing exercise at an intensity that exceeds the level of usual activity for 30 minutes three times a week should help to prevent bone loss in many adults.

More important is to avoid prolonged immobilization. The role of isometric exercises in patients with established osteoporosis is beneficial to avoid bone loss and control of falls. The effect of exercise on bone mass may be enhanced by calcium supplementation and the benefits from estrogen and exercise appear to be additive.

The phase of net bone loss is commonly thought to begin at or around the menopause but in fact starts earlier and is accelerated after the menopause. The rate of bone loss varies considerably among the population. Some cases with accelerated bone loss could be identified, namely "fast-losers", by bone-densitometry or biochemical markers. In this group and for those with already established osteopenia or osteoporosis by densitometric definition, a pharmacological approach is indicated and association of certain antiresorptive drugs, including estrogens, is advisable.

Several drugs have been shown to prevent or at least to decrease the rate of bone loss early after menopause. Calcium must be supplemented as aging is associated both with a reduced dietary intake and a relative malabsorption of calcium. Dietary calcium should therefore be evaluated and, if necessary, brought up to a daily intake of 1.000 mg in women on estrogen and 1.500 mg in those not on estrogens. Food and dietary products bestow enough calcium in healthy women but in some cases calcium preparations are necessary. The elemental content of calcium is important. The availability of calcium is greater with meals. Calcium supplements divided over the meals are not to exceed 500 mg. Prevention of eventual side-effects must be taken in consideration.

Calcitonin in pharmacological amounts is an inhibitor of bone resorption. Several studies confirm a decrease in vertebral fracture frequency, vertebral deformities and of the risk of hip fracture. 50 IU/day given by nasal spray for 5 days per week prevent bone loss at the spine after menopause. Larger doses might be required at cortical sites. New preparations and ways of administration will reduce inconvenient side-effects.

Bisphosphonates are now widely used for prevention of bone loss, not only in perimenopausal women but also in patients taking corticosteroids and other forms of secondary osteoporosis. Table 18.1 shows the regimens of bisphosphonates most frequently used and/or under study in human clinical trials. These doses prevent bone loss. The effects on fracture rate are discussed in Chapter 20.

A great variety of combinations, sequential and intermittent regimes, has been studied for prevention of osteoporosis. Ipriflavone, raloxifene, strontium salts may be of interest in the near future. In cases with associated arterial hypertension, thiazide diuretics, through its effect on renal tubular reabsorption of calcium, could be a good choice.

Table 18.1. Bisphosphonates to prevent bone loss in osteoporosis and/or under study in human clinical trials (Kanis, 1996)

Agent	Dose (mg)	Regimen
Etidronate*	400	2 weeks out of 12
Tiludrontate	50–200	7 days out of 28
Clodronate	800	Daily or daily every other month
Pamidronate	150	Daily or intermittent
Alendronate*	10	Daily
Ibandronate	2.5	Daily (also 5 mg 3 monthly i.v.)
Risedronate	5	Daily or 2 weeks on 2 weeks off

*given with calcium

Summary

Prevention includes control of strong risk factors early after menopause, such as different diseases, nutritional factors, smoking, alcohol excess, certain drugs and immobilization. The role of calcium intake and physical activity is stressed. Antiresorptive drugs, as calcitonins or bisphosphonates play a important role in preventing osteoporosis and bone fractures.

Suggested Reading

Dawson-Hughes B. (1995) Prevention. In: *Osteoporosis*. Riggs BL, Melton LJ III (eds) 2nd edn. Lippincott-Raven, Philadelphia pp. 335–350.

Kanis JA. (1996) *Osteoporosis*. Blackwell, Oxford pp. 148–167.

Woolf AD, St. John Dixon A. (1988) *Osteoporosis: A Clinical Guide*. Martin Dunitz, London pp. 146–154.

19

Prevention in Old Age: Pharmacologic and Non-Pharmacologic Strategies to Prevent Hip Fracture

Steven Boonen

Hip fractures among the elderly are a worldwide epidemic, and the number of these fractures is expected to rise dramatically as the populations age. In addition to high financial costs, femoral neck fractures are associated with high morbidity, high risk for long-term institutionalization, and increased risk of death. Considering the magnitude of the problem, any substantial reduction in the hip fracture burden depends on prevention. In view of the complex pathogenesis of hip fractures, preventive strategies should focus on the frequency of falling in the elderly as well as on the prevalence of compromised femoral integrity as a consequence of bone loss.

Ex vivo experiments on cadaveric specimens have indicated that over 90% of the variance in femoral failure load in a fall configuration can be predicted by measuring bone mineral density at the proximal femur, suggesting that the age-dependent decrease in bone mass is the most important cause of diminishing bone strength with aging and, therefore, of osteoporotic fracture risk. Consistent with this assumption, bone mineral density has been shown to associate significantly with hip fracture in prospective cohort studies.

The increase in hip fractures with age, however, is not fully accounted for by the decline in bone mineral density of the proximal femur: even after adjustment for bone density, each decade increase in age is still associated with a substantial increase in fracture risk in elderly women. Other factors, in addition to bone density, must therefore increase the susceptibility to hip fractures. These factors contribute to the risk of hip fracture in other ways, presumably by influencing qualitative characteristics of bone other than bone density or by affecting the incidence or impact of falls.

Targeting of Preventive Strategies

In addition to low bone mass, many potential risk factors for hip fracture, such as low body mass index, previous fractures, muscle weakness, impaired vision, cognitive impairment, a history of hyperthyroidism, use of long-acting sedatives, and physical inactivity have been identified in case-controlled and prospective studies. Although some of these factors act as least partly through effects on bone density, recent data indicate that numerous risk factors still exert significant effects on the risk of fracture after adjustment for bone density and that the assessment of risk factors and the measurement of bone density have complementary value for the prediction of hip fracture. In a prospective cohort study by Cummings et al. involving 9516 community-based women 65 years of age or older, women who had five or more risk factors (15% of the study population) had a probability of fracture in the next five years of about 10%, whereas the 47% of women with two or fewer risk factors had a probability of about 1%. Moreover, the incidence-ratio of hip fracture ranged from 1.1 (95% confidence interval 0.5–1.6) per 1000 woman-years among women with no more than two risk factors and normal bone density for their age to 27 (95% confidence interval 20–34) per 1000 woman-years among those with five or more risk factors and bone density in the lowest third of their age. These findings indicate that a small number of women with multiple risk factors and low bone density have an especially high risk. They account for a large proportion of hip fractures and should be the focus of intensive preventive efforts. While some risk factors may not be directly modifiable, their increased attributable risks suggest that targeting equivalently effective preventive efforts at these subgroups may result in a greater reduction in the rate of serious injury than a preventive program aimed at the overall elderly population. Moreover, the identification of several disparate risk factors, none with a large relative risk, supports the multifactorial nature of hip fracture and suggests that a multidimensional rather than a single, intervention strategy may result in the greatest risk reduction.

Pharmacologic Strategies to Prevent Hip Fracture

Even in women aged 80 years and over, bone density continues to be strongly associated with the risk of femoral fractures. Based on these and similar data, age-related fractures are considered to be primarily the consequence of bone loss and increased *bone fragility*. In line with this dominant view on fracture etiology, prevention studies have primarily focused on pharmacologic interventions to increase bone density of the femoral neck.

Prevention of Estrogen Deficiency-Induced Bone Loss at the Proximal Femur

The residual effects of estrogen deficiency-related bone loss (partially) account for the higher incidence of hip fractures in elderly women compared to elderly men, even though the rates of slow bone loss are similar. As a consequence of the combined effects of both types of bone loss, bone density of the femoral neck declines about 58% over a lifetime in women (39% in men), while density of the intertrochanteric region of the proximal femur falls about 53% (35% in men).

A significant effect of *estrogen substitution therapy*, initiated perimenopausally, on bone density, including mineral density at the proximal femur is well-documented. In women who receive lifelong therapy, bone density at 80 years may decrease by about 10% from bone density at menopause, as compared with a decline of about 30% in women who have never been treated. However, when estrogen substitution is discontinued, bone density declines at a rate similar to the perimenopausal one. About 10–15% of skeletal mass is estrogen-dependent, implying that this amount of bone is rapidly lost in postmenopausal women, perimenopausally if estrogen therapy is not initiated or later in life when estrogen substitution is discontinued. In a cross-sectional analysis involving 212 postmenopausal women (mean age 76 years) from the Framingham Study, Felson et al. reported on the long-term effect of postmenopausal estrogen substitution on bone density. Among women of 75 years old or older, even 10 or more years of past estrogen therapy were not associated with a significant effect on femoral bone density.

In line with these densitometric data, several cross-sectional studies have provided evidence to suggest that the protective effect of estrogen substitution on hip fracture incidence does not persist after discontinuation of the estrogen therapy. In a study by Weiss and co-workers involving 320 postmenopausal women and 567 age-matched controls, a decreased risk of fracture (0.43, 95% confidence interval 0.3 to 0.6) was evident only in case of *current* estrogen intake. Similar findings were reported in a retrospective cohort analysis of 2873 women in the Framingham Study. The adjusted relative risk in women who had taken estrogens within the previous 2 years was reduced to 0.34 (0.12 to 0.98). In contrast, past estrogen use was less protective (0.74, 0.49 to 1.14). Finally, the waning effect of postmenopausal estrogen therapy on senile osteoporosis was recently confirmed by a prospective cohort study involving 9704 ambulatory women 65 years of age or older. The relative risk for hip fracture tended to be lower among current users (0.60, 0.36 to 1.02) than among never-users. Previous use of estrogen, even for more than 10 years, had no substantial effect on fracture risk. To prevent hip fractures in old age, estrogen treatment may have to be initiated perimenopausally and continued indefinitely.

Prevention of Age-related Femoral Bone Loss

The cumulative response of a deficit in calcium intake and an age-related decline in calcium absorption, which is partially accounted for by vitamin D deficiency, is a negative calcium balance stimulating parathyroid hormone (PTH) secretion. Serum PTH has indeed been reported to show a significant, though limited, age-related increase. This age-associated increase in intact PTH is (partially) determined by the progressive decline in vitamin D [$25(OH)D_3$] status, suggesting that age is associated with mild secondary hyperparathyroidism necessary to maintain normal serum $1,25(OH)_2D_3$ concentrations. In addition, the ability of PTH to increase renal 1α-hydroxylase activity appears to diminish with age, possibly owing to diminished renal mass, and this may contribute to the age-associated increase in PTH.

In the concept of age-related (type II) osteoporosis, a key role has indeed been attributed to this vitamin D deficiency-related secondary hyperparathyroidism. In line with this concept, the increase in serum PTH with aging correlates directly with the increase in markers of bone turnover. High serum PTH levels resulting from low calcium intake and vitamin D deficiency are therefore likely to contribute to bone loss by inducing an age-related increase in activation frequency, i.e., the number of remodeling units activated. As there is already a net loss of bone within each remodeling cycle in the elderly and as PTH increases the birth of new remodeling units, the effect of secondary hyperparathyroidism will be to amplify the uncoupling between bone resorption and formation and to increase the amount of bone lost per unit time.

Effect of Calcium Substitution on Bone Loss and Fracture Risk

Much of the research on the effect on dietary calcium in the elderly has focused on the relationship of calcium intake to bone density rather than fracture and has yielded contradictory results. A more consistent relationship has emerged from several calcium supplementation trials, which generally have shown a small, but positive, effect of calcium on bone loss in older women. Fewer studies have examined the relationship between dietary calcium and hip fracture risk, and these have also produced conflicting results. However, most of these studies have used a case-control design. Recently, a number of prospective studies on the role of calcium in hip fracture risk have been published, and each has produced somewhat different results, possibly because of different ranges of dietary calcium, unstandardized dietary assessments, misclassification errors, and/or sampling variation due to fluctuating dietary intakes. In fact, only one prospective study to date has demonstrated a statistically significant protective effect of calcium in postmenopausal women, suggesting that there is no overall effect of dietary calcium on hip fracture risk. However, although not statistically significant, the finding of decreased relative risks in all other prospective studies indicates that further investigation may be warranted. In particular, future research should clarify if, and to what extent, calcium may be more effective in certain age subgroups of postmenopausal women. In this regard, recent data suggest that the effect of calcium may vary during menopause, being relatively ineffective in attenuating bone loss until late menopause. This issue is elucidated clearly in a study by Dawson-Hughes et al., in which, with the same investigational design, the same measurement methods, and the same calcium sources, a modest calcium supplement abolished age-related femoral bone loss in (vitamin D-replete) women 6 or more years postmenopausal, but was quite without effect in women within 0–5 years following menopause. Similarly, in a recent cohort study of non-institutionalized women aged 50–74 years, the age-adjusted risk of hip fracture was substantially reduced in the highest quartile of calcium intake compared to the lowest quartile, but only in the subgroup of women who were at least 6 years postmenopausal. In general, these evaluations of the relationship between calcium intake and fracture risk in elderly women are suggestive of a beneficial effect.

The effectiveness of calcium supplementation in suppressing hyperparathyroidism and reducing fracture incidence will depend on the dosage of the calcium supplement. While the optimal intake of calcium that is required to maximize PTH suppression remains to be established, the current recommended dietary allowance (RDA) of 800 mg per day in older subjects undoubtedly is inadequate. In fact, even in (vitamin D-replete) women with a daily intake of 800 mg of calcium, both parathyroid function and markers of bone remodeling are markedly elevated. In contrast, recent evidence suggests that women over age 65, maintained for 3 years on a calcium intake averaging 2400 mg per day, manifest not the values of PTH secretion and bone resorption typical for their age, but young adult normal values instead. The fact that secondary hyperparathyroidism is not prevented by a calcium intake approximating 800 mg per day (as recommended by the Food and Nutrition Board of the National Academy of Sciences), and that PTH levels can be returned to young normal values at a calcium intake well-above the current RDA is a clear indication of the inadequacy of the current 800 mg figure for the elderly and supports the recent recommendation of the National Institutes of Health Consensus Conference on Calcium Nutrition that elderly subjects should consume at least 1500 mg of calcium per day.

In addition to the dosage of the calcium supplement, timing of the administration may be important. Recent studies indicate that bone resorption is characterized by circadian variation, and the daily rhythm of PTH secretion of calcium intake is likely to be an important determinant of this rhythm. Attenuation of the circadian rhythm of bone resorption by oral calcium supplementation may therefore critically depend on the timing of the supplements. Consistent with this assumption, evening calcium supplementation abolishes the night-time increase in levels of PTH, attenuates the circadian rhythm of bone resorption, and reduces overall daily bone resorption in healthy premenopausal women. In contrast, morning calcium supplementation has no significant effect on the circadian rhythm of bone resorption. Although it remains to be established whether similar findings apply to older people, these data suggest that evening calcium supplementation may be required to suppress hyperparathyroidism-induced bone loss in the elderly.

Effect of Vitamin D Substitution on Bone Loss and Fracture Risk

To test the effect of vitamin D on the incidence of hip and other osteoporotic fractures in elderly women, large-scale intervention studies have recently been reported. In a prospective, randomized study in 3270 elderly women with a mean calcium intake of 500 mg per day and a mean serum $25(OH)D_3$ of 15 ng/mL, Chapuy and co-workers reported that, compared to placebo, supplementation with cholecalciferol (800 IU per day) and calcium (1.2 g per day) increased bone mineral density at the proximal femur and reduced the risk of hip fracture significantly (Table 19.1).

After 18 months, femoral bone density had increased 2.7% in women who were given the supplement and declined 4.6% in placebo recipients. Women who received cholecalciferol and calcium had a 25% decrease in the incidence of hip fractures and other peripheral fractures. Moreover, support was provided (increased serum 25(OH)D$_3$ and decreased serum PTH concentrations) for a biochemical mechanism of this effect. However, these strong findings must be tempered by the wide age range of the 3270 subjects studied (69–106 years of age), the high dropout rates (30% withdrew for reasons other than death) and the lack of a factorial design that would allow the relative merits of each of the supplements to be determined.

Table 19.1. Effects of Vitamin D$_3$ and calcium supplementation on the number of fractures in elderly women.

	Vitamin D$_3$ (800 IU) and Calcium (1.2 g)	Placebo	P Value
Active-treatment analysis			
Number of women	1208	1168	–
All nonvertebral fractures	151	204	0.020
Hip fractures	73	103	0.040
Intention-to-treat analysis			
Number of women	1387	1403	–
All nonvertebral fractures	160	215	<0.001
Hip fractures	80	110	0.004

Chapuy et al., *N Engl J Med* 1992.

Lips et al., on the other hand, recently conducted a prospective double-blind trial in 2578 elderly men and women (mean age 80 years) to study the effect of cholecalciferol substitution (400 IU per day). No calcium supplement was used. While the participants in the Chapuy trial were mainly residents of nursing homes, about 40% of the participants in the Lips study lived independently. Mean daily calcium intake was 1,000 mg and mean serum 25(OH)D$_3$ level 10 ng/mL. Despite a significant increase in femoral mineral density of 2.2% after 2 years, no effect on fracture incidence was noted during a median follow-up of 42 months.

It is unlikely that the higher dose of vitamin D in the Chapuy study is responsible for the difference in results. The additional increase in serum 25(OH) D$_3$ when using a 800 IU dose is negligible, which is confirmed by the similar increase of serum 25(OH) D$_3$ in both studies. Although mean baseline serum 25(OH) D$_3$ and age were similar, the dietary calcium intake was much lower in the Chapuy study, which may account for the higher baseline serum PTH levels and the subsequently greater reduction after supplementation. In fact, the decrease in serum PTH concentration in a sample of the Chapuy study was about 50% after calcium and vitamin D treatment, whereas this concentration decreased only 15% in a nonrandom sample from the Lips trial after vitamin D supplementation. These changes in parathyroid activity suggest that the calcium supplement contributed substantially to the observed effects in the Chapuy trial. Thus, the effect of vitamin D supplementation might be greater when a calcium supplement is also used. In addition, the effect of vitamin D substitution on the incidence of fractures may only be apparent in an older, frailer population than the one studied by Lips. In line with this assumption, recent retrospective data have provided further evidence that the use of vitamin D supplements is not associated with a significant decrease in overall risk of hip fracture in community-based women, supporting the concept that vitamin D might be targeted optimally to the frail elderly institutionalized population.

Non-pharmacologic Strategies to Prevent Hip Fracture

About 1% of falls cause hip fracture and about 5% result in any type of fracture. *In vitro* data on the relationship between bone mineral density and fracture load have indicated that an increase of more than 20% in femoral neck mineral density would be required to raise the mean fracture load to the level of the impact loads from a fall on the hip. However, controlled trials of pharmacologic interventions have demonstrated increases of only a few per cent in femoral neck density emphasizing the continuing need for intervention strategies that focus on fall prevention and/or reduction in fall impact.

Prevention of Falls

Over 90% of hip fractures have been documented to be the result of falls. The annual incidence of falls among elderly persons living in the community increases from 30% after 65 years of age to 40% among those over the age of 80. Falls are even more common in the institutionalized elderly, which may contribute to the fact that institutionalized elderly people are not protected from sustaining a hip fracture. Although some falls have a single cause, the predisposition to fall may, rather, result from the accumulated effect of multiple factors.

Falls are complex, multifactorial events, and this may partially explain the fact that they have been proven remarkably resistant to prevention. Recently, however, Tinetti et al. reported that an intensive multifactorial intervention strategy could be used to decrease the incidence of falls (Table 19.2). The study population consisted of noninstitutionalized men and women who were at least 70 years of age and who had at least one or more selected risk factors for falling. In the subjects assigned to intervention, standardized intervention protocols were used for each identified risk factor. Three types of intervention were applied: adjustment in medications, behavioral instructions and exercise programs. During 12 months of follow-up, 35% of the intervention group fell, as compared with 47% of the control group, corresponding with an adjusted incidence-rate ratio for falling of 0.69 (95% confidence interval 0.52–0.90). In addition, the proportion of persons who had the targeted risk factors for falling was reduced in the intervention group, suggesting that risk factor modification contributed to the decreased occurrence of falls. Similarly, combined data from a number of recent trials have demonstrated that certain exercise programs significantly reduce the fall incidence ratio in elderly patients.

Table 19.2. Multifactorial intervention strategy to reduce the risk of falling among elderly people.

Risk factors	Intervention
◆ Postural hypotension	Behavioral recommendations; decrease in dosage, discontinuation, or substitution for medications that may contribute to hypotension
◆ Use of any benzodiazepine or other sedative-hypnotic agent	Education about the appropriate use of sedative-hypnotic agents; nonpharmaco-logic treatment of sleep problems; tapering and discontinuation of medications
◆ Use of 4 prescription medications	Review of medications with primary physician
◆ Inability to transfer safely to bath-tub or toilet	Training in transfer skills; environmental alterations, such as grab bars or raised toilet seats
◆ Environmental hazards for falls or tripping	Appropriate changes, such as removal of hazards, safer furniture (correct height, more stable), installation of structures such as grab bars or handrails on stairs
◆ Any impairment in gait	Gait training; use of an appropriate assistive device; balance or strengthening exercises if indicated
◆ Any impairment in transfer skills or balance	Balance exercises; training in transfer skills if indicated; environmental alterations
◆ Impairment in muscle strength	Resistance training

Tinetti et al., *N Engl J Med* 1994.

However, the degree to which the effects of these interventions can be generalized will need to be determined in other settings. Moreover, no effect of the strategies studied was documented on hip fracture incidence. While multifactorial fall prevention efforts have demonstrated moderate reductions in fall incidence, such programs are expensive and potentially inefficient. In fact, none of the studies individually or collectively in any meta-analysis had an effect on injurious falls. The critical question of the efficacy of preventive strategies for fall injuries will therefore have to await clinical trials specifically designed for that purpose and specifically targeted on selected subgroups.

Reduction of Impact of Falls

The loads required to fracture the isolated elderly femur *in vitro* are significantly (an order of magnitude) smaller than estimates of the potential energy generated during a typical fall from standing height. Even at rates of load applied during a typical fall, the estimated impact force on the hip is 35% greater than the average femoral fracture load. These experimental findings suggest that the energy transmitted during falling and impact, rather than bone strength, may be the dominant factor in the biomechanics of fracture of the hip. The energy transmitted to the proximal femur during a fall may vary considerably, as it is determined by the impact energy created by the fall and the energy absorption capacity of the trochanteric soft tissue.

An *external protective device*, designed to divert the impact energy from the greater trochanter, has been shown to significantly reduce the energy transmitted to the proximal femur and may substantially reduce the risk of hip fracture in elderly individuals. In a randomized prospective trial by Lauritzen and co-workers, application of a polypropylene device to nursing home residents was associated with a relative risk of femoral fracture of 0.44 (95% confidence interval 0.21 to 0.94). The diversion of the impact away from the greater trochanter did not result in an increase in non-hip fractures. In addition, all subjects in the intervention group who sustained a fracture failed to use their protectors at the time of the injury.

Conclusion

By any standard, osteoporosis is one of the most important diseases encountered in geriatric practice. The complexity of the pathogenesis of hip fractures implies the need for a multifaceted strategy of prevention. Although many risk factors for senile osteoporosis are potentially preventable or reversible with targeted interventions, the beneficial effects of most strategies have not yet been adequately documented, indicating the need for additional long-term controlled studies.

Summary

- Strategies for the prevention of hip fracture should focus on the frequency of falling as well as on the prevalence of compromised femoral integrity as a consequence of bone loss.
- Given the high prevalence of falls among the elderly, a performance-oriented functional assessment should be targeted at all patients over 75 years of age. As the risk of falling increases with the number of risk factors, risk may be reduced by modifying even a few contributing factors.
- Recent intervention studies have indicated the need to provide adequate supply of both calcium and vitamin D (1500 mg and 400 IU daily, respectively), in particular to the frail elderly institutionalized population.

Suggested Reading

Boonen S, Dequeker J. (1996) Strategies for the prevention of senile (type II) osteoporosis. *J Int Med* 239: 383–91.

Chapuy M, Arlot M, Duboeuf F et al. (1992) Vitamin D_3 and calcium to prevent hip fractures in elderly women. *N Engl J Med* 327: 1637–42.

Cummings SR, Nevitt MC, Browner WS et al. (1995) Risk factors for hip fracture in white women. *N Eng J Med* 332: 767–73.

Felson D, Zhang Y, Hannan M, Kiel D, Wilson P, Anderson J. (1993) The effect of postmenopausal estrogen therapy on bone density in elderly women. *N Engl J Med* 329: 1141–6.

Lips P, Graafmans W, Ooms M et al. (1996) Vitamin D supplementation and fracture incidence in elderly persons. *Ann Intern Med* 124: 400–6.

McKane WR, Khosla S, Egan KS et al. (1996) Role of calcium intake in modulating age-related increases in parathyroid function and bone resorption. *J Clin Endocrinol Metab* 81: 1699–1703.

Lauritzen JB, Petersen MM, Lund B. (1993) Effect of external hip protectors on hip fractures. *Lancet* 341: 11–13.

Tinetti M, Baker D, McAvay G et al. (1994) A multifactorial intervention to reduce the risk of falling among elderly people in the community. *N Engl J Med* 331: 821–7.

20

Treatment of Osteoporosis

Henry G. Bone

Once the diagnosis of osteoporosis is established, a plan of medical intervention should be formulated, taking into account the severity of the osteoporosis, any contributory causes, other medical conditions which may influence treatment, and the circumstances of the patient.

The evaluation of the patient for contributory causes of decreased bone mass, and appropriate specific intervention when such conditions are found, is essential to successful treatment of the disorder. Obviously, medical disorders such as Cushing's disease, myeloma or gluten enteropathy, should be addressed directly. More common are subtle abnormalities affecting bone and mineral metabolism. Specifically, many patients with osteoporosis are found to have nutritional deficiencies, or impaired calcium and/or vitamin D absorption. It is also not uncommon for patients with osteoporosis to have renal calcium wasting. Such patients may have a personal or family history of urolithiasis. One or more contributory factors may be present in as many as one-fourth or more of patients with osteoporosis, and may be even more common in patients whose osteoporosis is especially severe or premature.

In patients in whom abnormalities of calcium metabolism have been excluded or corrected, contemporary treatment is directed at altering the balance of bone remodeling, generally by suppressing bone resorption. In most cases this is accomplished with hormone replacement therapy or non-hormonal antiresorptive agents. However, the role of mechanical loading must not be forgotten. Regular weight bearing exercise is an essential part of any successful regimen.

Treatment of Disorders of Calcium Metabolism

Nutritional Deficiencies

Inadequate dietary calcium and vitamin D intake are common, especially in the elderly or institutionalized patient. The effectiveness of supplementation of calcium and vitamin D in such patients has been well demonstrated to alleviate such deficiency states, with a consequent reduction in fracture rate. Clinical studies of calcium administration, and the evaluation of placebo-control group subjects receiving calcium supplements in many clinical trials, have demonstrated the ability of adequate calcium and vitamin D nutrition to at least stabilize the bone mass in many patients. Typical recommendations include 1,500 milligrams of elemental calcium daily, in divided dosage, and four hundred to eight hundred international units of vitamin D per day, depending on the patient's sunlight exposure. Various calcium preparations are available including tablets, capsules, solutions and fortified beverages. Some patients find calcium supplements constipating. In such cases, dairy products, calcium-enriched beverages (e.g. orange juice) and aqueous solutions are apt to be better tolerated. Stool softeners and generous water intake are also important. Alternatives to calcium carbonate may be better tolerated by patients who are bothered by release of carbon dioxide gas. The effectiveness of nutritional therapy can be judged by measurement of the twenty-four urine calcium excretion, which should increase from the subnormal pre-treatment levels typical of deficiency states to the normal range within a few months on the supplements. It is also useful to measure 25-hydroxyvitamin D levels to assure adequacy of vitamin D treatment. Target serum 25-hydroxyvitamin D levels are at least 20 ng/ml and preferably 30 ng/ml.

Impaired Calcium Absorption

More problematic are patients who are unable to absorb adequate amounts of calcium and/or vitamin D even when usually adequate amounts are taken by mouth. On careful evaluation, some of these patients will be found to have gluten enteropathy, although such patients will often have little in the way of gastrointestinal symptoms (in contrast to patients whose celiac disease is diagnosed earlier). These patients may respond to gluten-free diets but will usually require extra calcium and vitamin D, as recovery of absorptive function may be slow and incomplete. Administration of parenteral vitamin D or oral calcifediol (25-hydroxyvitamin D) generally will be adequate to provide normal circulating vitamin D levels in such patients, but small amounts of extra calcitriol (1,25-dihydroxyvitamin D) supplementation may be useful when the gut surface is not adequate to respond to normal vitamin D levels. Other patients will have impaired absorption due to a variety of identifiable conditions (for example Crohn's disease) which may be amenable to medical intervention. When the underlying condition can not be completely corrected, extra calcium supplementation and parenteral administration of vitamin D or oral administration of its more potent metabolites may be required. It is particularly important to monitor the urinary calcium and oxalate excretion in patients with fat malabsorption because such patients may have hyperoxaluria, and may be prone to urolithiasis even in the presence of normal urinary calcium excretion. In such patients, special efforts to reduce the fat intake and control dietary oxalate will be important, and calcium adminstration may help to control oxalate absorption.

It is also fairly common to find impaired renal 1-alpha hydroxylation of vitamin D in older patients with osteoporosis, especially in patients with mild, often sub-clinical, deterioration of renal function. Such patients may not be adequately treated with ordinary supplements and may also require treatment with a potent vitamin D metabolite to correct the calcium malabsorption problem. A further group of elderly osteoporotic patients have apparently normal vitamin

D metabolism or have received compensatory therapy, and nevertheless may have poor absorption of calcium. The mechanism of this age-related impairment of calcium absorption is undetermined, but if increased amounts and frequency of calcium prove ineffective, cautious use of calcitriol may help. Great care must be used in the prescribing of calcitriol as it can cause hypercalciuria and/or hypercalcemia in as many as one-third of patients receiving just 0.5 micrograms per day. When used in osteoporosis patients it should be given cautiously starting with 0.25 mcg daily. The serum and 24-hour urine calcium levels must be monitored after about two months on treatment and two to three times per year thereafter. Dosage of the calcitriol and calcium can then be adjusted. Other potent vitamin D analogues may be less dangerous but care must still be taken to adjust the dose to the individual patient. When possible, calcifediol should be used, leaving the final regulatory step, 1-alpha hydroxylation, intact. Calcitriol acts by stimulating intestinal calcium transport and it also directly suppresses parathyroid hormone at the glandular level. However, calcitriol is in addition an extremely potent stimulant to bone *resorption*, and therefore is truly a double-edged therapeutic sword. Generally in cases where the use of potent vitamin D metabolites is considered, specialist consultation is appropriate.

Renal Calcium Wasting

This condition, which has traditionally been associated with urolithiasis, may have an increased frequency in the elderly population, in which it appears to be associated with osteoporosis. These patients will have excessive 24-hour urine calcium excretion, often with high-normal to mildly elevated parathyroid hormone levels, as well as elevated fasting urinary calcium/creatinine ratios. As long as the patient maintains a low sodium intake, oral treatment with thiazide diuretics or indapamide is generally effective in suppressing the renal calcium excretion into the normal range, thereby correcting the associated mild secondary hyperparathyroidism, and restoring calcium balance. It is critically important to measure sodium excretion in such patients prior to and on therapy so that the role of sodium in the generation of the hypercalciuria can be appreciated in the individual case. The usual considerations associated with the use of diuretics, such as potassium balance, apply in hypercalciuric patients as well as any other.

Pharmacotherapeutic Interventions in Bone Remodeling

Most currently available drugs for osteoporosis act primarily by controlling bone resorption. The dominant mechanism for early increases in bone mass in patients receiving anti-resorptive drugs is the *remodeling transient* effect, whereby the bone remodeling space is reduced, with the reduction in remodeling space being seen as an increase in bone mass. In addition to decreasing bone mass, excessive rates of bone resorption may contribute to fragility by perforating trabeculae and creating weak points which may become fracture sites. Thus control of resorption may provide benefits in addition to increased bone mass.

Estrogen Replacement Therapy

Estrogen replacement therapy influences bone and mineral metabolism in several respects. Firstly, excessive bone resorption is decreased. This appears to be the dominant mechanism of action of estrogen in patients with rapid postmenopausal bone loss. Secondly, intestinal calcium absorption is enhanced. Thirdly, there may be favorable effects on bone formation mediated by direct estrogen effects on osteoblasts and/or a favorable effect on local production of growth factors within bone. Use of estrogen does not eliminate the need for adequate calcium and vitamin D.

Mechanisms of Action

Available estrogen preparations all appear to have essentially similar effects on bone metabolism, varying mainly with respect to potency and therefore dosage requirements. Although some progestins may have modest effects on bone metabolism, these are much less important than the effects of the estrogen with which the progestins are administered. Estrogens clearly reduce the excessive bone resorption associated with estrogen deficiency. This acceleration of bone resorption is probably due to elevation of tissue levels of pro-osteolytic cytokines in bone. There is increasing evidence that the anti-osteolytic effects of estrogen are mediated at least partly by suppression of excessive levels of IL-6, perhaps IL-1, and possibly other cytokines which are increased in estrogen deficient women. Serum 25-hydroxyvitamin D, and calcitriol levels are increased by estrogen administration, which may explain the finding of improved calcium absorption in estrogen treated patients. The increase in total serum levels of vitamin D metabolites is in large part due to increased serum vitamin D-binding protein levels. However, *free* calcitriol levels have been demonstrated to increase as well. Finally, there may be beneficial effects of estrogen on stromal cells and osteoblasts. These effects and their significance are much less well defined, but the presence of estrogen receptors in those cells has been demonstrated.

Dosage and Administration

Perhaps the most important issue in successful estrogen therapy is regulation of the dosage. Proper regulation of the estrogen dosage is essential to achieving both efficacy and good tolerability. Various trials have been conducted to identify efficacious dosages. In such trials, many patients have a good result on doses lower than those required to produce a benefit in every patient. This is more likely to reflect variations in absorption and metabolism of the medications than true variation in target tissue responsiveness. Most of the anti-resorptive effect of estrogen is achieved at steady state serum estradiol levels over about 50-60 pg/ml. Levels of greater than 130 pg/ml are rarely, if ever, required for control of postmenopausal vasomotor symptoms. Clinical dose-response relationships for the other estrogen effects on bone and mineral metabolism are not well characterized, but clinically effective dosages have been identified for the commonly used estrogens. Typically recommended dosages for common estrogens include estradiol, 0.5–2.0 mg orally per day or 50–100 mcg daily by transdermal administration. Conjugated equine estrogens are usually effective at 0.625 mg p.o. daily. It is noteworthy that in patients taking conjugated equine estrogens, absorption and cleavage of estrone sulfate, followed by the metabolism of estrone to estradiol accounts for the production of the most active steroid and allows for a number of points of potential variation in metabolism of this very widely used medication.

In those women who do not have vasomotor symptoms, a dosage near the low end of the effective range for a particular estrogen preparation may be used as a starting dosage in order to minimize mastodynia and other symptoms. After a month or two, the dosage can then be titrated up using serum estradiol levels and markers of bone turnover to achieve an effective dosage on an individualized basis. It is desirable to achieve mid-normal *premenopausal* indices of bone resorption. In contrast, women with clinical vasomotor symptoms will generally require a somewhat larger starting dosage in order to relieve those symptoms promptly. The same principles of titration on the effects on bone metabolism may still be employed. It should not be assumed that single dosage of estrogen is optimal for all patients although the popular dosages are typically effective in a large percentage of women. Although in the past many physicians have prescribed estrogen on a twenty-five days per month basis or some other cyclic approach, currently used estrogen dosages are generally designed to achieve early follicular phase levels of estrogen in the serum and do not require cyclic administration. Therefore, the estrogen is usually given on a continuous or daily basis.

Endometrial Effects

In patients who have not undergone hysterectomy, management of the uterine effects of estrogen is of great importance in achieving a successful long-term treatment program. The major objective is to prevent endometrial hyperplasia and endometrial carcinoma, and it is extremely important to minimize unscheduled bleeding. Progestins may be used on a cyclic basis to induce a regular shedding of the endometrial lining. This is an approach that has been shown to have a protective effect on the endometrium and has been successfully used for many years. In typical regimens the estrogen is administered daily, and the progestin is administered for twelve to fourteen days of each cycle, with bleeding expected at about day ten to twelve. Many older women especially find regular menstruation annoying, so regimens have been designed to minimize bleeding. The continuous combined treatment regimen is now widely employed. In this program, not only is the estrogen given on a daily basis, but so is the progestin. The purpose is to prevent the stimulation and proliferation of the endometrial lining. This approach is effective in a majority of patients, if both the patient and the physician are prepared for a few months of irregular bleeding, which often occurs. However, perhaps one-third of patients will not achieve amenorrhea within six months. Most such patients will switch to regular cyclic therapy, so the bleeding will at least be predictable and scheduled, or they may choose a non-estrogenic anti-resorptive treatment.

Risk-Benefit Assessment

A major concern about estrogen is, of course, the question of its role in the creation of excessive risk for breast cancer. Although even meta-analyses of this risk vary in their conclusions, it does seem that there is little if any increase in risk at moderate doses of estrogen given for up to five years or perhaps somewhat more, but there may be increasing risk with higher doses and longer-term treatment. On the other hand, there is considerable evidence of major favorable effects of estrogen on cardiovascular risk. With careful surveillance for breast cancer using modern mammographic techniques, the risk to the patient is probably much less than the benefit obtained from prevention of cardiovascular morbidity, as well as the prevention of osteoporosis and minimization of urogenital atrophy. There is also increasing evidence that there may be a favorable effect on cerebral function in women taking estrogen. Thus, for women with no specific contraindication to estrogen therapy, the risk-benefit analysis is generally very favorable. The anticipated introduction of selective estrogen receptor modulators (see below) may eventually have an important impact on the use of estrogen.

Androgen Therapy

Androgens are, of course, highly appropriate therapy for osteoporosis in testosterone deficient men. Both transdermal and intramuscular depot formulations are useful. Androgens are sometimes used in the treatment of osteoporosis in women, but their usefulness is greatly limited by their virilizing effects and unfavorable influence on lipid metabolism.

Non-estrogen Anti-resorptive Agents

The Calcitonins

Calcitonins are 32 amino acid peptides which act by means of specific receptors on osteoclasts to suppress the activity of those cells. Thus calcitonins are in principle extremely specific and selective physiological anti-resorptive agents. The safety record of calcitonin has been outstanding, with virtually no history of major long term adverse effects. Until recently the usual route of administration was by injection, but nasal calcitonin sprays have been introduced which deliver therapeutically adequate dosage of calcitonin for most patients. A number of clinical trials have demonstrated a modestly favorable effect on bone mass in patients with osteoporosis. In some studies, this effect has been concentrated in patients with particularly high rates of bone turnover and much less pronounced in patients with modest rates of bone turnover. In addition to the modest effect on bone mass, there is some evidence for a beneficial effect on fracture rate.

However, the evidence concerning antifracture efficacy is less definite than for some other medications.

Salmon calcitonin has been administered as a subcutaneous injection in a typical dosage of 50 iu daily. This medication has an excellent safety record, but can cause flushing and/or nausea. Initiating therapy with much lower dosages (10-20 iu) and gradually increasing as tolerated, appears to reduce the adverse effects. One possible advantage of injected calcitonin is relief of skeletal pain which is reported by some patients. This effect is neither well understood nor altogether predictable, but can be useful, especially in the period after compression fractures. The nasal calcitonin spray has achieved much better tolerability than was the case with the injections. A typical regimen of nasal calcitonin is 200 international units sprayed daily in alternating nostrils. This probably delivers about 25-50 international units in the average patient. It is extremely important for patients on calcitonin to have adequate calcium and vitamin D intake and absorption since calcitonin can cause a calciuric effect and may actually result in secondary hyperparathyroidism if adequate calcium and vitamin D are not present. Monitoring of the anti-resorptive effect of calcitonin is particularly important, and measurement of baseline and on-treatment levels of urinary collagen metabolites or other measurements of bone resorption/turnover is important so that therapy can be adjusted in order to achieve an optimal result.

Bisphosphonates

The geminal bisphosphonates are pyrophosphate analogues which are widely used in the treatment of various bone and mineral disorders including osteoporosis. The pioneer drug in this class was etidronate, an effective anti-resorptive drug which causes defective mineralization at about the same dosage as that which controls bone resorption. This became a clinically significant problem at the higher doses employed for Paget's disease of bone and was a concern in the management of osteoporosis as well. Therefore a regimen was devised in which etidronate was administered cyclically for two weeks out of every three months. Calcium is administered during the eleven weeks off etidronate, but is avoided during the period of treatment with etidronate because it prevents the absorption of the medication. This strategy appears to have minimized the clinical significance of the mineralization defect, although focal osteomalacia has been described in biopsy specimens from clinical trials. In clinical trials, etidronate was shown to increase bone mineral density. However, the definitive phase III studies failed to demonstrate consistent and convincing evidence of overall antifracture efficacy, although there was some evidence for a favorable effect in a high risk subgroup.

Subsequent generations of bisphosphonates have been designed to enhance anti-resorptive potency and diminish the relative potency of the anti-mineralizing effect. Pamidronate has been used in a variety of bone disorders and was shown to be effective in the treatment of osteoporosis, but problems with tolerability in a more recent formulation has impaired its introduction into clinical use as an oral agent. Intravenous pamidronate has been shown to be useful in the treatment of osteoporosis, especially that associated with transplantation. Clodronate has not been used extensively in the treatment of osteoporosis, although it has similar potency to etidronate without the mineralization defect. At the time of writing, the bisphosphonate with the greatest clinical importance for the treatment of osteoporosis is alendronate. This aminobisphosphonate is much more potent than etidronate and somewhat more potent than pamidronate, and does not have any clinically significant adverse affect on matrix mineralization. A very extensive program of clinical trials has been conducted, demonstrating a substantial increase in bone mass on treatment. This occurs rapidly in the first six to twelve months, as would be expected due to the bone remodeling transient effect, but appears to continue into the third year at least. Favorable effects on bone mass have been noted not only in the spine but also in the femur, radius and total body measurements when compared with placebo-treated subjects. In a large, carefully conducted study, alendronate given as 5 mg per day for two years and 10 mg per day for the third year, resulted in a reduction in fracture rates of about 50% in osteoporotic women with low bone mass and at least one vertebral compression fracture prior to study entry. Similar percentages of fracture reduction were noted for both the spine and long bones. Even more impressive was the reduction by approximately 90% in the number of women having second vertebral fractures during the study. One potential adverse effect of this generally well-tolerated medication is esophageal irritation, particularly in patients with reflux or other esophageal dysfunction. This was not a common problem in clinical trials, in which patients with severe gastroesophageal reflux were usually excluded. It is essential that the medication be taken with water only and that a period of at least one-half hour elapse prior to food being ingested, otherwise absorption of the medication may be very substantially impaired. As with all anti-resorptive medications, a background of adequate calcium and vitamin D nutrition is essential to therapeutic success with bisphosphonates. Other bisphosphonates in clinical development for osteoporosis include risedronate, tiludronate, and ibandronate. These medications may be appearing on the clinical horizon within the next few years. The mechanisms of action are substantially similar, and the points of differentiation amongst them will be expected to emerge in the course of clinical trials.

Fluoride

Fluoride is the only stimulant of bone formation that is used extensively in clinical practice. After more than thirty years of evaluation and use, its role is still controversial. It has been well demonstrated that fluoride stimulates formation of bone. However, fluoride is also incorporated into the bone mineral structure forming fluoroapatite. This appears to alter the mechanical properties of bone in fluoride-treated animals and humans. Mechanical strength testing has shown that there is a progressive loss of strength as fluoride content in bone increases. In addition, fluoride can cause osteomalacia and formation of woven bone. Thus there is persistent concern about the integrity of the relationship between bone mass and bone strength in fluoride-treated patients. In consideration of this problem, prospective, double-blind, placebo-controlled clinical trials of 75 mg of fluoride daily were conducted at two large medical centers. In both of these trials, fluoride increased bone mass as measured radiographically, but failed to improve fracture rates, and in fact there were numerically more fractures seen in the fluoride treated group than in the control subjects. It has been suggested that the dosage of fluoride employed in those trials was excessive. Additional studies have been performed at lower dosages. In one relatively small study, using a proprietary slow-release fluoride preparation, an apparent reduction in fractures was reported. Caution must be used in interpreting and generalizing the results of this small study, however. In a recent, much larger multi-center study, employing a similar dosage of fluoride in a different formulation, no improvement in fracture rate was achieved. It has been suggested that a very narrow therapeutic window may exist in which fluoride can be administered safely and effectively, but this has not been adequately corroborated to overcome the concerns raised by a long history of preclinical and clinical studies. In view of the unfavorable experience with fluoride in several well controlled studies, recommendation of "slow-release" or other preparations of fluoride for general use must await corroboration by favorable results in large multi-center trials. At the time of writing, it seems that fluoride should be used with great caution, if at all. It should probably never be used in patients with a relative deficit of cortical bone, although it may have a limited place in the treatment of predominantly axial osteoporosis.

On the Horizon and Beyond

Estrogen Agonists/Antagonists

Following the discovery that tamoxifen has a mitigating effect on bone loss, a number of other mixed estrogen antagonists have been investigated as anti-osteoporosis agents. These agents are also known as selective estrogen receptor modulators (SERMs). Preliminary results with these agents suggest that they are capable of producing an estrogen-like effect on bone resorption in estrogen-deficient animals and women and may have an estrogen-like effect on lipid profiles as well. On the other hand, they appear to have an antiestrogenic effect on breast and uterine tissue. Thus these agents may have a very attractive profile of effects for the prevention and treatment of osteoporosis in postmenopausal women who do not require estrogen for symptom control. Long-term studies of the safety and efficacy of these agents are ongoing, but core clinical trials for raloxifene are nearly complete at the time of writing. It seems likely that slightly different profiles will emerge for different SERMs. This may result in a very advantageous situation from the standpoint of patients and physicians, if the drug profile can be matched to individual patient requirements. Conceivably, urogenital symptoms of estrogen deficiency might be managed with low-dose intravaginal estrogen in patients who take SERMs for their systemic affects. At the present time, it appears that women in the early postmenopausal period who are troubled with vasomotor symptoms will still require true estrogens.

Other Agents

Parathyroid hormone, parathyroid hormone-related peptide and their analogues are especially interesting because of their ability to stimulate cancellous bone formation. However, increased cortical bone resorption remains a problem at this time. Roles for IGF-I and perhaps other growth factors have also been suggested. These agents will remain investigational for the foreseeable future. Ipriflavone and tibolone are also under investigation but their role has not been established. Advances in the understanding of the molecular and cell biology of bone are expected to provide more opportunities for intervention in the next few years.

Exercise

Regular, weight-bearing exercise, such as walking, is essential to the maintenance of skeletal mass. Thirty minutes of walking three or four times weekly should prevent loss of bone due to lack of mechanical loading. The possible role of resistance training with heavy weights in the treatment of osteoporosis remains to be established. Patients with back pain due to kyphosis caused by compression deformities usually find that a well-designed, correctly performed program of exercises for the improvement of posture, strengthening of the back and abdominal muscles and relief of muscle spasm, will provide greater pain relief than analgesics and promote an enhanced sense of well-being.

Summary and Conclusions

A well-planned program of treatment for osteoporosis depends on correction of all underlying nutritional and physiologic abnormalities. Superimposed on this physiologic approach is a strategy of controlling bone resorption in order to achieve a more favorable balance between resorption and formation. The selection of therapy in an individual patient must take into account that patient's other particular needs and characteristics. For instance, a woman with severe vasomotor symptoms will generally require estrogen replacement in one form or another, while a woman who has had a breast malignancy will probably not be a good candidate for estrogen, and must use an alternative anti-resorptive. Long-term therapy with estrogen seems to be well tolerated and effective, although increasing attention must be paid to the risk of breast cancer with high doses and protracted treatment. Similarly, the approved non-estrogen anti-resorptive agents seem to be safe and effective, although very long-term treatment experience is not as yet available. At the time of writing we do not have satisfactory stimulants of bone formation to repair the imbalance from the other side of the equation. Although fluoride may be useful in carefully selected cases, serious concerns about its detrimental effects on bone strength and mineralization remain. Individualized therapy based on normalized physiology remains the cornerstone of the successful program of intervention.

Suggested Reading

Black DM, Cummings SR, Karpf DB, Cauley JA, Thmpson DE, Nevitt MC, Bauer DC, Genant HK, Haskell WL, Marcus R, Ott SM, Torner JC, Quandt SA, Reiss TF, Ensrud KE. (1996) Randomised trial of effect of alendronate on risk of fracture in women with existing vertebral fractures. Fracture Intervention Trial Research Group. *Lancet* 348(9041): 1535-41.

Chapuy MC, Arlot ME, Duboeuf F, Brun J, Crouzet B, Arnaud S, Delmas P, Meunier PH. (1992) Vitamin D3 and calcium to prevent hip fractures in elderly women. *N Eng J Med* 327(No.23): 1637-1641.

Cummings SR. (1991) Evaluation of benefits and risks of postmenopausal hormone therapy. *Am J Med* 91(5B):14S-18S.

Dawson-Hughes B, Dallal GE, Krall EA, Sadowski L, Sahyoun N, Tannenbaum S. (1990) A conrolled trial of the effect of calcium supplementation on bone density in postmenopausal women. *N Eng J Med* 323:878-883.

Devogelaer JP, Broll H, Correa-Rotter R, Cumming DC, De Deuxchaisnes CN, Geusens P, Hosking D, Jaeger P, Kaufman JM, Leite M, Leon J, Liberman U, Menkes CJ, Meunier PJ, Reid I, Rodriguez J, Romanowicz A, Seeman E, Vermeulen A, Hirsch LJ, Lombardi A, Plezia K, Santora AC, Yates AJ, Yuan W. (1996) Oral alendronate induces progressive increases in bone mass of the spine, hip, and total body over 3 years in postmenopausal women with osteoporosis. *Bone* 18(2):141-50.

Draper MW, Flowers DE, Huster WJ, Neild JA, Harper KD, Arnaud C. (1996) A controlled trial of raloxifene (LY139481) HCI: Impact on bone turnover and serum lipid profile in healthy postmenopausal women. *J Bone Miner Res* 11(6):835-42.

Francis RM, Peacock M, Taylor GA, et al. (1984) Calcium malabsorption in elderly women with vertebral fractures: Evidence for resistance to the action of vitamin D metabolites on the bowel. *Clin Sci* 66:103-107.

Gallagher JC, Riggs BL, Eisman J, Hamstra A, Arnaud SB, DeLuca HF. (1979) Intestinal Ca absorption and serum vitamin D metabolites in normal subjects and osteoporotic patients. *J Clin Invest* 64:729-736.

Gallagher JC, Riggs BL, DeLuca HF. Effect of estrogen on calcium absorption and serum vitamin D metabolites in postmenopausal osteoporosis. *J Clin Endocrinol Metab* 51(6):1359-1364.

Garnero P, Delmas PD. (1996) New developments in biochemical markers for osteoporosis. *Calcif Tiss Int* 59 Suppl 1:S2-9.

Harris ST, Watts NB, Jackson RD, Genant HK, Wasnich RD, Ross P, Miller PD, Licata AA, Chesnut CH. (1993) Four-year study of intermittent cyclic etidronate treatment of postmenopausal osteoporosis: three years of blinded therapy followed by one year of open therapy. *Am J Med* 95(6):557-67.

Lufkin EG, Wahner HW, OiFallon WM, Hodgson SF, Kotowicz MA, Lane AW, Judd HL, Caplan RH, Riggs BL. (1992) Treatment of postmenopausal osteoporosis with transdermal estrogen. *Ann Intern Med* 117 (1):1-9.

Mattson LA, Cullberg G, Samsioe G. (1982) Evaluation of a continuous oestrogen-progestogen regimen for climacteric complaints. *Maturitas* 95-102.

McKane WR, Khosla S, Egan KS, Robins SP, Burritt MF, Riggs BL. (1996) Role of calcium intake in modulating age-related increases in parathyroid function and bone resorption. *J Clin Endocrinol Metab* 81(5):1699-703.

Meunier PJ, Sebert J-L, Reginster J-Y, Briancon D, Appelboom T, Netter P, Loeb G, Rouillon A, Barry S, Evreux J-C, Avouac B, Marchandise X, FAVOStudy Group. (in press) Flouride salts do not better prevent vertebral fractures than calcium-vitamin D in postmenopausal osteoporosis: The FAVOStudy. *Osteoporosis Int*

Need AG, Horowitz M, Philcox JC, Nordin BC. (1985) 1,25-Dihydroxycholecalciferol and calcium therapy in osteoporosis with calcium malabsorption. Dose response relationship of calcium absorption and indices of bone turnover. *Mineral & Electrolyte Metabolism* 11(1):35-40.

Nordin BEC, Need AG, Morris HA, Horowitz M, Robertson WG. (1991) Evidence for a renal calcium leak in postmenopausal women. *J Clin Endocrinol Metab* 72:401-407.

Overgaard K, Hansen MA, Jensen SB, Christiansen C. (1992) Effect of salcatonin given intranasally on bone mass and fracture rates in established osteoporosis: a dose-response study. *BMJ* 305(6853):556-61.

Recker RR, Hinders S, Davies KM, Heaney RP, Stegman MR, Lappe JM, Kimmel DB. (1996) Correcting calcium nutritional deficiency prevents spine fractures in elderly women. *J Bone Miner Res* 11(12):1961-6.

Riggs BL, Hodgson SF, O'Fallon WM, Chao EYS, Wahner HW, Muhs JM, Cedel SL, Melton LJ. (1990) Effect of fluoride treatment on the fracture rate in postmenopausal women with osteoporosis. *N Engl J Med* 322:802-809.

Stampfer MJ, Colditz GA, Willett WC, Manson JE, Rosner B, Speizer FE, Hennekens CH. (1991) Postmenopausal estrogen therapy and cardiovascular disease. *N Engl J Med* 325(11):756-762.

Thiebaud D, Burckhardt P, Malchior J, Eckert P, Jacquet AF Schnyder P, Gobelet C. (1994) Two years effectiveness of intravenous pamidronate (APD) versus oral fluoride for osteoporosis occuring in the postmenopause. *Osteoporosis Int* 4:76-83.

21

Surgical Therapy of Fractures

Karl J. Obrant & Olof Johnell

Osteoporotic fracture, also called fragility fracture, is defined as a fracture occurring with increasing frequency with age and more commonly in women. There are numerous types of such fractures, the most serious one being the hip fracture. Also, wrist fracture, vertebral fracture or fracture of the proximal humerus are frequently sustained by osteoporotic women.

Wrist Fracture

The wrist fracture is the most common osteoporotic fracture. The typical patient is a postmenopausal 65-year old woman living independently. The fracture is usually sustained outdoors and in increasing numbers in icy conditions. Therefore, in an orthopaedic department such as the authors' place of work, representing a recruitment area of 250,000 inhabitants and situated in Northern Europe, the number of such fractures is usually one or two every day, with a record of 55 fractures in one day! The fracture is sustained when falling with the arm extended, in an attempt to protect the body with the palm taking the impact. A dorsal and radial compression of the distal radius appears (Colles' fracture). In fewer than 10% of the cases there is a volar angulation instead (Smith fracture).

The Colles' fracture is reduced by applying traction on the first and second digits and thereafter volar forced angulation. A plaster-of-Paris cast is applied on the dorsoradial aspect of the forearm (Figure 21.1).

It is important to make allowance for the fingers as well as the elbow to be able to move freely, to instruct the patient to use the arm and hand as much as possible and also to carry the arm in a position as high as possible in order to avoid swelling and immobilization atrophy. After reduction, an X-ray examination is performed to ascertain that the fracture is in an acceptable position in the plaster. Another X-ray examination is performed after 10 days in order to detect those 5–10% of fractures that re-dislocate in spite of being fixated. For fractures without complications 4 weeks in a plaster cast is usually long enough. Thereafter free mobilization is allowed. For the fractures which initially can not be reduced or those which have re-dislocated after 10 days, some kind of primary or secondary operative procedure may be necessary. In young individuals with high demands on their wrist an exploration of the fracture system and internal fixation may become necessary.

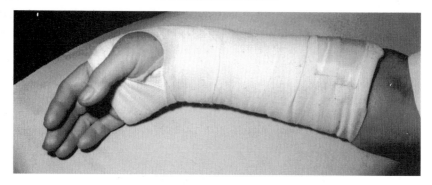

Figure 21.1. Colles' fractures are usually treated by applying a short plaster-of-Paris cast on the dorsoradial aspect of the forearm. Four weeks of immobilization are usually enough for fracture healing.

The outcome after Colles' fracture is usually regarded as good, but 25% of patients will, even three years after the fracture event, experience a loss of strength and some stiffness. There are women who suffer a re-fracture of their distal radius once or even several times. Each such event results in an additional impairment of the function of the wrist.

Shoulder Fracture

Fracture of the surgical neck of the proximal humerus is not uncommon in older women. The reason for sustaining this type of fracture is usually an impact force directly onto the shoulder. Mostly, this fracture is not very dislocated, making a conservative treatment regimen feasible. Only seldom is the fracture severely dislocated or comminuted, in which case an open reduction with or without osteosynthesis is necessary. In a "four-fragment" type of fracture there is no hope for fracture healing and normal function of the shoulder. In younger individuals with this type of fracture a joint arthroplasty should be considered.

In uncomplicated cases of this type of fracture, a few weeks of immobilization in "straps-and-bandages" is advisable and alleviates pain. After this short period, free mobilization is allowed, but the services of a physiotherapist may be necessary. The rehabilitation period is usually extended over several months, and the end-result is not always favourable in terms of range of motion. Most patients, however, will eventually be free of pain.

Vertebral Fracture

The epidemiology of vertebral fracture is poorly understood, since up to 50% of these fractures may be subclinical and the individual affected will not seek medical advice. The fracture, subclinical or not, may appear after any insignificant trauma. In severely osteoporotic women an unusual or severe cough may be sufficient to fracture one or several vertebrae. Vertebral fractures sustained after low energy trauma are hardly ever defined as unstable and do not result in complications on the spinal canal. Therefore, in more than 99% of these cases conservative, non-operative treatment is advocated. There is hardly ever need for specific orthopaedic regimens for these patients. After a few days of rest it is advisable that the patient mobilizes herself as much as possible in order to avoid further demineralization, which inevitably occurs after a fracture and especially after long-time immobilization. Mild analgesics and prescription for an orthopaedic corset or crutches may alleviate the patient's symptoms. Outcome studies after vertebral fractures have usually found that there is a social impairment and persistent backpain, especially in those individuals who have two or several fractured vertebrae.

Hip Fracture

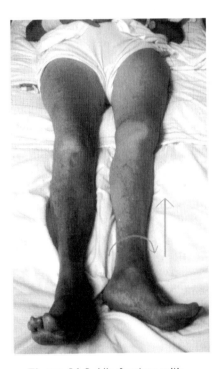

Figure 21.2. Hip fracture with typical shortening and outward rotation of the affected limb.

Hip fracture patients usually present at the emergency room after falling with immediate impact on the lateral aspect of the hip followed by inability to stand or walk. In typical cases the extremity is rotated outward and shortened (Figure 21.2). It is impossible from a clinical examination to judge whether a fracture is intracapsular (femoral neck fracture) or extracapsular (trochanteric fracture). After an X-ray examination the exact diagnosis can be set. The distinction between the two types of fracture is important since the operative treatment and the outcome varies considerably. If surgical facilities are available to undertake the operation promptly there is no need for pin traction, but if the patient has to wait several hours or maybe days for surgery an applied pin traction can be of value since it may alleviate pain in the hip region. In general, there is consensus that surgery is the treatment of choice for both femoral neck fracture and trochanteric hip fracture, although in some very unusual cases of impacted fractures or when the patient has severely impaired general health, conservative treatment may be advisable.

Femoral Neck Fracture

Since the middle of this century almost all of these fractures have been internally fixated, in all countries in the Western World. Such a fixation can be performed with different devices, of which there are hundreds on this flourishing market. The interpretation of this situation should be that no device is better than another. Common for all of them, however, is that there is a very high rate of postoperative complication. The main complications occurring are, early secondary displacement, pseudarthrosis and femoral head necrosis. Especially in primarily displaced femoral neck fractures, the complication rate is high, and approximately half of the patients complain of symptoms of restricted walking ability or continuous pain leading to re-operation for about every third patient. The secondary operation performed is then often an arthroplasty.

Because of the high number of operative failures after internal fixation of these fractures, the orthopaedic community has turned more and more to performing primary arthroplasties on these patients. The decision as to whether this arthroplasty should be a hemi-arthroplasty replacing only the femoral head, or a total joint replacement is based on the age of the patient and her general physical status. The rationale for this is that total arthroplasties are considered to stay intact for longer than hemi-arthroplasties. The latter operation, on the other hand, is a considerably smaller surgical trauma for the patient, and is therefore advocated in the very old or frail patient with a prognosis indicating limited mobility. Also after arthroplasty, however, the complication rate is not negligible. The main complication is dislocation of the artificial joint, which will lead to an inevitable reduction under general anaesthesia once or several times, and in a few cases also a re-operation. The frequency of such dislocations is higher in these patients than in patients operated because of osteoarthritis, because hip fracture patients are often senile and do not cooperate postoperatively. Also, the decreased muscular mass in such elderly individuals will promote joint laxity, which will therefore lead to an increased risk of dislocations.

There are very few prospective, randomized studies where internal osteosynthesis has been compared to joint replacement. From the few that exist, however, it would appear that arthroplasty is to be preferred, at least in severely dislocated fractures.

Trochanteric Hip Fracture

Despite the fact that this fracture engages more bone than does the femoral neck fracture, it poses a much smaller problem. The operative treatment performed at most centers today is an internal fixation with a sliding screw introduced into the femoral neck and femoral head, and which in turn is allowed to slide in a cylindrical plate itself attached to the femur by separate screws. This concept allows for impaction of the fracture fragment when the patient puts his weight on the leg. Fracture healing is therefore enhanced. In spite of some shortening of the fractured extremity after healing, there are no long-term complications associated with this type of fracture. The short-term complications are few and hardly more than 5% of the patients will have to be re-operated.

Rehabilitation after Hip Fracture

Regardless of whether internal fixation or joint arthroplasty has been performed, the patient is allowed to walk and to put weight on the fractured leg the day after operation. Only in severely comminuted fractures or in fractures where the operative procedure has not been good should there be a restriction on weight bearing. The time when these patients can return to their original accommodation varies considerably.

Summary

The orthopaedic treatment for most fragility fractures is generally uncontroversial, except for minor details. For the hip fracture, and especially the femoral neck fracture, on the other hand, there are great controversies due to the high complication rate, whatever treatment modality we have chosen. There is an ongoing effort, with large, prospective studies, to try to solve these controversies. Independent of the outcome of these studies, there is consensus that the treatment of hip fracture will remain a challenge.

22

Osteoporosis in Men

Ego Seeman

In 1990, about 30% of the 1.7 million hip fractures worldwide occurred in men. The age specific incidence of hip fractures is increasing. By the year 2025 the number of hip fractures in men will be similar to the numbers seen in women now and will be compounded by the greater numbers seen in women (Figure 22.1). The morbidity and mortality of hip fractures is three times higher in men than women. The prevalence of spine fractures is similar in men and women, around 10–20% of persons over 65 years of age. Whether the fractures are the result of trauma in youth or underlying bone fragility is uncertain. In men, the incidence of forearm fractures is low and remains so throughout old age.

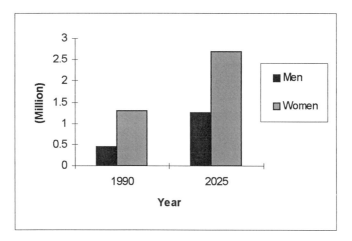

Figure 22.1. By the year 2025, the number of men with hip fractures will be similar to the number of women with hip fractures in 1990 (adapted from Cooper et al).

Pathogenesis: Reduced Bone Gain and Increased Bone Loss

A low peak bone mineral density (BMD), excessive bone loss or both mechanisms contribute to the reduced BMD found in men with fractures. Peak bone *mass* is greater in men than in women because men have bigger bones (Figure 22.2). Peak volumetric bone *density* is the same in men and women —

the amount of bone in the bone is the same in men and women. The amount of trabecular bone loss is similar in men and women but perforation in women (due to increased resorption) results in loss of connectivity while trabecular thinning (due to reduced bone formation) in men results in maintenance of the connectivity. Men lose less cortical bone than women because subperiosteal cortical bone formation is greater in men than in women while endosteal resorption is greater in women than in men.

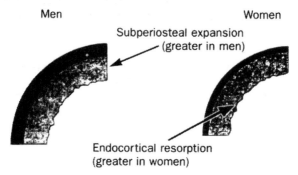

Figure 22.2. Cortical bone loss occurs by endosteal thinning in women and men. The cortical thinning in men is less than in women because of compensatory periosteal bone deposition which maintains the bending strength of bone.

Fracture incidence is lower in men than women because in men the diameter of the vertebral bodies and long bones is greater at maturity, bone loss relative to peak is less (10 versus 25%), trabecular loss occurs by thinning not perforation (Figure 22.3) and cortical thinning by endosteal resorption is offset by periosteal deposition.

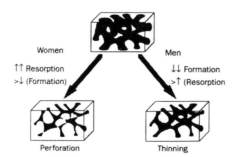

Figure 22.3. Trabecular thinning occurs in men because reduced bone formation is the main mechanism responsible for bone loss. Trabecular perforation occurs in women because of the increased bone turnover associated with menopause.

Sex Hormone Deficiency, Secondary Osteoporosis and Risk Factors

Testosterone falls with age due to a decreased Leydig cell number, changes in hypothalamic-pituitary function and coexistent illness. This is usually not accompanied by a rise in gonadotrophins. Risk factors for fractures include excessive alcohol intake, tobacco use, inactivity, leanness, low calcium intake, and reduced strength. Drug therapy such as corticosteroids, anticonvulsants, heparin, excessive thyroid hormone replacement may cause bone loss (Table 22.1).

Table 22.1. Osteoporosis in men: Assessment of men presenting with spine or hip fractures: Differential diagnosis

Common
♦ usually idiopathic
♦ hypogonadism
      - idiopathic (normal gonadotrophins)
      - testicular failure (elevated gonadotrophins)
      - alcoholism
♦ alcoholism (without hypogonadism)
♦ myeloma (secretory and nonsecretory)

Uncommon
♦ hypogonadism secondary to
      - Klinefelter syndrome
      - prolactinoma
      - kallman's syndrome
      - haemochromatosis
      - hyperprolactinaemia
      - pituitary tumour
      - anorexia nervosa
♦ malabsorption, adult onset celiac disease
♦ Cushing's dyndrome
♦ primary hyperparathyroidism
♦ idiopathic hypercalciuria
♦ mastocytosis
♦ thyrotoxicosis

Fractures may be the presenting, and sometimes the only, clinical feature of diseases including multiple myeloma (secretory and nonsecretory), adult onset celiac disease, Cushing's syndrome, primary hyperparathyroidism, idiopathic hypercalciuria, mastocytosis and others. Each of these illnesses must be considered in the differential diagnosis of men presenting with fractures (Figure 22.4). Many illnesses associated with osteoporosis have effects on gonadal function, a treatable cause of bone loss (idiopathic hypogonadism, pituitary tumors, Klinefelter syndrome, hyperprolactinemia, anorexia nervosa, excessive exercise, haemochromatosis, exogenous corticosteroids) (Table 22.2).

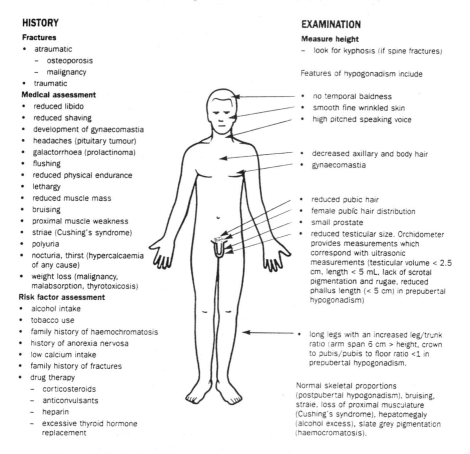

HISTORY

Fractures
- atraumatic
  - osteoporosis
  - malignancy
- traumatic

Medical assessment
- reduced libido
- reduced shaving
- development of gynaecomastia
- headaches (pituitary tumour)
- galactorrhoea (prolactinoma)
- flushing
- reduced physical endurance
- lethargy
- reduced muscle mass
- bruising
- proximal muscle weakness
- striae (Cushing's syndrome)
- polyuria
- nocturia, thirst (hypercalcaemia of any cause)
- weight loss (malignancy, malabsorption, thyrotoxicosis)

Risk factor assessment
- alcohol intake
- tobacco use
- family history of haemochromatosis
- history of anorexia nervosa
- low calcium intake
- family history of fractures
- drug therapy
  - corticosteroids
  - anticonvulsants
  - heparin
  - excessive thyroid hormone replacement

EXAMINATION

Measure height
- look for kyphosis (if spine fractures)

Features of hypogonadism include

- no temporal baldness
- smooth fine wrinkled skin
- high pitched speaking voice

- decreased axillary and body hair
- gynaecomastia

- reduced pubic hair
- female pubic hair distribution
- small prostate
- reduced testicular size. Orchidometer provides measurements which correspond with ultrasonic measurements (testicular volume < 2.5 cm, length < 5 mL, lack of scrotal pigmentation and rugae, reduced phallus length (< 5 cm) in prepubertal hypogonadism)

- long legs with an increased leg/trunk ratio (arm span 6 cm > height, crown to pubis/pubis to floor ratio <1 in prepubertal hypogonadism.

Normal skeletal proportions (postpubertal hypogonadism), bruising, straie, loss of proximal musculature (Cushing's syndrome), hepatomegaly (alcohol excess), slate grey pigmentation (haemocromatosis).

Figure 22.4. Medical history and clinical examination in the differential diagnosis of osteoporosis in men.

Falls

No fall, no hip fractures. Falls among 2793 respondents over 65 years was 28%; 19% in men and 34% in women during 12 months. Sedative use, cognitive impairment, lower extremity disability and palmomental reflex are risk factors for falls. In 232 men aged 35 to 96 years with hip fracture from moderate trauma (compared to controls). The risk of hip fracture was increased two-fold overall in the presence of thyroidectomy, gastric resection, pernicious anemia, and chronic bronchitis and almost seven-fold in the presence of risk factors for falls such as hemiplegia, Parkinsonism, dementia, blindness, and vertigo. These two classes of risk factors together accounted for 72% of the hip fractures.

Table 22.2. Investigations in men with osteoporosis.

Test	Explanation or suspected condition
Testosterone	SHBG*, T/SHBG ratio
Follicle stimulating hormone and luteinizing hormone	are usually inappropriately normal in patients with reduced testosterone. This may indicate the presence of a pituitary tumour, but usually not. The inappropriately normal levels suggest age-related decrease in hypothalamic pituitary function.
Prolactin	prolactinoma
Full blood examination	anaemia?, myeloma, malabsorption
Protein electrophoresis and immunoelectrophoresis, Bence-Jones protein	myeloma
Bone marrow biopsy	may be needed to diagnose nonsecretory myeloma
Calcium	- low (malabsorption, vitamin D deficiency) - high (primary hyperparathyroidism, myeloma)
Phosphate	-low in osteomalacia, primary hyperparathyroidism
Alkaline phosphatase	sometimes elevated (after fracture, coexistent Paget's disease)
24 hour urine calcium excretion	seen in osteoporosis in young men
Creatinine clearance	
screening PSA**	should be done when androgen therapy is administered although there are still no guidelines as to how frequently this should be done.

* SHBG = Sex hormone binding globulin

** PSA = prostate-specific antigen

Prevention and Treatment

Patients with painful fractures require reassurance that the pain is temporary. Relief of pain can be achieved with frequent analgesia, massage, physiotherapy and hot baths. Correction of risk factors is indicated (alcohol excess, tobacco use). Exercise is unlikely to increase BMD, it may prevent further bone loss.

Increasing Peak BMD and Preventing Bone Loss

The prevention of fractures in men involves attention to risk and protective factors influencing bone peak BMD, bone loss and falls. A 10–30% higher peak

Suggested Reading

Cooper C, Atkinson EJ, O'Fallon WM, Melton LJ III. (1992) Incidence of clinically diagnosed vertebral fractures: A population-based study in Rochester, Minnesota, 1985–1989. *J Bone Miner Res* 7(2): 221–227.

Cooper C, Campion G, Melton LJ. (1992) Hip fractures in the elderly: A world-wide projection. *Osteoporosis Int* 2: 285–289.

Davies KM, Stegman MR, Heaney RP, Recker RR. (1996) Prevalence and severity of vertebral fracture: The Saunders County Bone Quality Study. *Osteoporosis Int* 2: 160–165.

Jackson JA, Kleerekoper M. (1990) Osteoporosis in men: diagnosis, pathophysiology, and prevention. *Medicine* 69: 1347–152.

Poór G, Atkinson EJ, Lewallen DG, O'Fallon WM, Melton LJ III. (1995) Age-related hip fractures in men: clinical spectrum and short-term outcomes. *Osteoporosis Int* 5: 419–26.

Seeman E. (1995) The dilemma of osteoporosis in men. *Am J Med* 98(Suppl 1A): 75S–87S.

23

Corticosteroid-induced Osteoporosis

Vasi Naganathan & Philip N. Sambrook

Pathophysiology

Abstract

Corticosteroids are thought to cause bone loss by a combination of inhibitory effects on bone formation and enhanced bone resorption, with the inhibitory effects on bone formation appearing to be most important.

For the most part, the decreased bone formation is due to direct effects on cells of the osteoblastic lineage although indirect effects related to sex steroid production are also important. Corticosteroids have complex actions on gene expression in bone cells dependent on the stage of osteoblast growth and differentiation. Corticosteroids decrease cell replication and repress type I collagen gene expression by the osteoblast by decreasing the rates of transcription and destabilizing $\alpha1(I)$ collagen mRNA. Corticosteroids have complex and unique effects on collagen degradation and regulate the synthesis of matrix metalloproteinases. In addition to direct actions on the collagen gene, corticosteroid effects on skeletal cells may be indirect and involve effects on the synthesis, release, receptor binding or binding proteins of locally produced growth factors. Corticosteroids decrease IGF-I synthesis in osteoblasts by transcription mechanisms and inhibit IGF-II receptor expression in osteoblasts.

Corticosteroids also decrease net intestinal absorption of calcium and increase urinary phosphate and calcium loss by direct effects on the kidney, contributing to secondary hyperparathyroidism and hence increased bone resorption.

It is generally considered that the majority of corticosteroid bone loss occurs in the initial 12–24 months of therapy and with chronic low dose therapy lesser loss is observed. The effect of corticosteroids is most apparent in regions of the skeleton with a high trabecular bone content, with fractures most commonly occurring in the spine and ribs.

Prevention

Corticosteroid effects on bone metabolism are reflected in marked changes in biochemical measures of bone turnover but at present there is no reliable way of predicting by such markers which patients will lose bone on corticosteroids. A bone density measurement remains the best predictor of risk of fracture and should be performed in patients starting high dose, long term corticosteroids as well as an x-ray of the thoracic and lumbar spine. If the bone density measurement reveals a reduced value or the spinal x-ray reveals a prior vertebral fracture, prophylaxis becomes most important. Currently only the bisphosphonates and the active vitamin D metabolites have evidence to support their efficacy for prophylaxis.

Bisphosphonates are analogues of pyrophosphate that bind to hydroxyapatite at sites of bone remodeling. They inhibit bone resorption primarily, and several bisphosphonates including etidronate, pamidronate, alendronate, tiludronate and residronate are available in various countries. At this time, only etidronate has been studied as a preventive agent in corticosteroid osteoporosis. In one small study in women with temporal arteritis commencing corticosteroids, the 10 who were randomized to cyclical etidronate exhibited no spinal bone loss compared to the 10 calcium treated patients. These data are encouraging but further prevention studies with newer more potent bisphosphonates are required.

The use of vitamin D in corticosteroid bone loss became popular following early studies, but these studies, which were not randomized, measured forearm rather than spinal bone density as their primary efficacy endpoint and, most importantly, were not primary prevention in design but rather conducted in patients on chronic corticosteroids with so called "established" osteoporosis.

More recent are the results of a prevention study comparing calcium 1000 mg daily plus vitamin D (50,000 units weekly) with placebo over 3 years. There was no statistically significant difference in spinal bone loss between calcium/vitamin D and placebo and the amount of bone loss observed at the spine after 12 months with the calcium/vitamin D combination was similar to that seen in the calcium alone treated control groups in two other recent prevention studies. Thus the use of calciferols as prophylactic agents remains uncertain.

Although the term vitamin D is sometimes used to encompass both the calciferols and calcitriol, this is misleading since calcitriol has quite a distinct therapeutic profile. Calcitriol is the active hormonal form of vitamin D, 1,25 dihydroxy-vitamin D. A recent study examined the effect of calcitriol as a preventative agent in a large randomized double blind controlled trial with spine bone density as the primary endpoint. Patients treated with calcium alone lost bone at the lumbar spine (−4.3% per year) whereas those treated with either calcitriol or calcitriol plus calcitonin lost bone at a much reduced rate (−1.3% and −0.2% per year respectively). There was no statistically significant difference between the two calcitriol groups, whereas both groups were significantly different from the calcium group. The mean daily dose of calcitriol used was 0.6 μg. A recent study with 1-alpha hydroxy vitamin D (alphacalcidol) confirms that the active vitamin D analogues have efficacy in prevention of bone loss in patients starting corticosteroids.

Treatment of Corticosteroid Osteoporosis

The first principle of treatment of corticosteroid induced bone loss is to use the lowest possible dose of corticosteroids. Corticosteroid osteoporosis may be partially reversible and whenever possible corticosteroids should be withdrawn. For patients with established corticosteroid osteoporosis on chronic therapy, numerous therapies have been studied including calcium, vitamin D metabolites, estrogen, bisphosphonates and calcitonin.

Although calcium supplements have been shown to decrease biochemical markers of bone resorption in corticosteroid treated patients, recent randomized controlled trials in patients starting corticosteroids where calcium was used as the control therapy suggest calcium at best offers only partial protection. Consequently, whilst an adequate calcium intake should be recommended, calcium alone probably does not have a major role to play in prevention or treatment of corticosteroid bone loss.

With regard to vitamin D, early studies suggested a role in the treatment of chronic corticosteroid users, but only the forearm site was studied. A recent study of calcium plus vitamin D_3 (500 IU/day) appears to confirm a benefit in patients with rheumatoid arthritis treated with chronic low dose corticosteroids, amounting to about a 2% difference compared to placebo. However there were some methodological problems with this study including that half of the baseline values of anteroposterior spinal bone density were estimated from lateral scans, not directly measured. Moreover the small rise in bone density may have largely been a "remodeling transient" whereby the increase was due to filling of bone spaces undergoing active remodeling.

Hypogonadism is commonly seen in males and females treated with corticosteroids suggesting a role for hormone replacement therapy. The combination of estrogen and progestogen therapy increased bone mass over one year in one small open study of post menopausal women with asthma on chronic corticosteroids and a randomized controlled trial of the effect of estrogen replacement therapy in rheumatoid arthritis reported a small benefit of treatment at the lumbar spine over two years in a subgroup of patients receiving low dose corticosteroids. Based on these studies, it is recommended that post menopausal women taking glucocorticoids should receive estrogen replacement if there are no contra-indications. No randomized trials have been performed in corticosteroid treated premenopausal women and in those with normal menstrual cycles, hormone treatment is inappropriate, although in woman with irregular menstrual cycles, use of the oral contraceptive may be indicated. In males, there has only been one study in a small number of asthmatics chronically treated with corticosteroids which showed a benefit with testosterone therapy at the spine but not the hip after 12 months of monthly injections. Accordingly, if the serum testosterone level is low in males, consideration should be given to the use of testosterone therapy in patients established on corticosteroids.

With respect to the bisphosphonates, a study in patients with corticosteroid dependent chronic obstructive airways disease treated with oral pamidronate demonstrated a significant increase at the lumbar spine over 2 years and several open studies suggest efficacy for cyclic etidronate in chronic corticosteroid users. It is reasonable to assume that the newer, more potent bisphosphonates will be similarly active in corticosteroid osteoporosis and currently there are several trials ongoing with these new generation bisphosphonates which will address this issue directly. However, because of the long skeletal retention, bisphosphonates are not normally used in treatment of younger individuals.

Calcitonin has been studied in patients starting corticosteroids and receiving chronic corticosteroids with varying results. A study in chronic corticosteroid users did show apparent benefit from calcitonin at the spine, but in two recent prevention studies, there was no statistically significant additional benefit of adding calcitonin to calcitriol or cholecalciferol.

Summary

Corticosteroids are widely used in the treatment of patients with chronic inflammatory diseases. Since the most rapid bone loss occurs in the first 12–24 months after commencing high dose corticosteroids, it is important to consider two different therapeutic situations, (a) prevention in patients starting corticosteroids and (b) treatment of patients on chronic corticosteroids who will already have some significant degree of corticosteroid related bone loss.

An adequate calcium intake is recommended and any contributing factors to osteoporosis should be treated. A bone density will give information about the future risk of osteoporotic fracture and the need for active pharmacological treatment. Patients commencing high dose long term corticosteroid therapy should be treated prophylactically with active vitamin D metabolites (alphacalcidol or calcitriol) or a bisphosphonate and the treatment may need to be continued for 1–2 years. Patients on chronic corticosteroids may improve their bone density by treatment with vitamin D metabolites (including the calciferols) and bisphosphonates. In post menopausal women, concomitant use of estrogen replacement therapy is also appropriate. In a patient on long-term therapy it is important to review the need for continuing treatment or the possibility of dosage reduction.

Suggested Reading

Hall GM, Daniels M, Doyle DV et al. (1994) The effect of hormone replacement therapy on bone mass in rheumatoid arthritis treated with and without steroids. *Arthritis and Rheumatism* 37: 1499–1505.

Mulder H, Struys A. (1994) Intermittent cyclical etidronate in the prevention of corticosteroid induced bone loss. *Br J Rheumatology* 33: 348–350.

Reid IR, Wattie DJ, Evans MC, Stapleton JP. (1996) Testosterone therapy in glucocorticoid treated men. *Arch Intern Med* 156: 1173–77.

Sambrook PN, Birmingham J, Kelly PJ et al. (1993) Prevention of corticosteroid osteoporosis; a comparison of calcium, calcitriol and calcitonin. *N Engl J Med* 328: 1747–52.

Sambrook PN, Jones G. (1995) Corticosteroid osteoporosis. *Br J Rheumatology* 34: 8–12.

24

Tumor-induced Osteolysis

Jean-Jacques Body

Some Important Clinical Aspects

The skeleton is the most common site of metastatic disease in breast and prostate cancer and the site of first distant relapse in almost one half of the patients with breast cancer. The most common sites of bone metastases are, in decreasing order, the thoracolumbar spine, the pelvis, the lower limbs, the upper limbs and the skull. On the other hand, multiple myeloma is almost always characterized by multiple lytic lesions, which constitute the hallmark of the disease although myeloma can also present as diffuse osteoporosis.

Tumor-induced osteolysis (TIO) of breast cancer is the source of a considerable morbidity, including pain, long bone fractures in 10–20%, and tumor-induced hypercalcemia (TIH) in 10–15% of the cases, although this last "classical" figure is certainly less nowadays because of the use of bisphosphonates. The median survival after first relapse in bone is close to 2 years compared to 3 months after first relapse in liver, which implies that the clinical burden induced by breast cancer-induced osteolysis is enormous. Metastatic skeletal disease actually accounts for the largest component of hospital costs in cancer patients.

A review of endocrine and chemotherapy trials suggests that patients with metastatic bone disease have a lower response rate to antineoplastic therapy than patients with soft tissue or visceral metastases. Low response rates in bone are actually probably artefactual due to the poor sensitivity of our current assessment methods. Symptom evaluation, measurement of tumor markers and of biochemical parameters of bone turnover should be more investigated for early assessment of bone response.

Pathophysiology of Tumor-induced Osteolysis: Rationale for the Use of Bisphosphonates

The propensity of breast cancer cells to metastasize in bone could notably be due to the rich supply of relevant growth factors present in the skeletal microenvironment, which can increase breast cancer cell growth. Bone destruction itself is essentially mediated by osteoclast activation rather than by direct osteolytic effects of metastatic cancer cells, although osteoblasts or immune cells could also be important target cells for the action of secretory products from various tumors.

Many studies have established the essential role of a parathormone-like substance, named parathyroid hormone-like protein (PTHrP) in all types of cancer hypercalcemia. The nature of the tumoral factor(s) responsible for osteoclastic activation in the complex process of TIO remains unknown, but recent data indicate that PTHrP could here too play an essential role. PTHrP-like substances are thus expressed by about 60% of human breast tumors and breast cancers metastasizing to the skeleton produce PTHrP more frequently than the tumors metastasizing to non-osseous sites. Local production of PTHrP and of other osteolytic factors such as TGFs by cancer cells in bone would stimulate osteoclastic bone resorption, partly through the osteoblasts, whose proliferation would also be inhibited, impairing the bone repair process. Such factors also induce osteoclast differentiation of hematopoietic stem cells and/or activate mature osteoclasts already present in bone. Increased osteoclast activity will then cause local foci of osteolysis, which could further stimulate cancer cells proliferation. These data indicate that it is rational to target bone-resorbing cells for the treatment and perhaps in the future the prevention of bone metastases.

Bisphosphonates are potent inhibitors of bone resorption. Their mechanism of action is complex and it is probable that several mechanisms are operative, the relative importance of each being a function of the chemical structure of the compound. Bisphosphonates localize preferentially to sites of active bone resorption and they can directly inhibit the activity of mature osteoclasts. The recruitment of osteoclasts could also be reduced, especially by aminobisphosphonates. Recent findings suggest that osteoblasts, or at least those lining the bone surface, could be the essential target cells for bisphosphonates with secondary effects on the osteoclasts, probably through a change in the secretion of an inhibitor of osteoclast recruitment. The relative importance of this osteoblast-dependent inhibitory activity of bisphosphonates compared to a direct inhibition of osteoclast activity remains to be determined. Whatever their precise mechanism of action, bisphosphonates have opened the way for a noncytotoxic medical treatment of bone metastases.

Bisphosphonates for the Treatment of Tumor-induced Osteolysis and its Complications

Tumor-induced Hypercalcemia (TIH)

The introduction of bisphosphonates has dramatically changed the therapeutic management of cancer hypercalcemia, whether of paraneoplastic origin or due to bone metastases. The superiority of pamidronate over etidronate, clodronate, mithramycin and calcitonin for the treatment of TIH has been demonstrated in several prospective comparative trials.

Rehydration (generally 2–3 litres of saline or its equivalent over 24–36 hrs) remains an essential therapeutic step but clodronate and pamidronate have supplanted all other compounds. A single-day 1500 mg infusion of clodronate is the most convenient way to administer that compound but it is less efficient than a 90-mg pamidronate infusion (generally infused over 3–4 hrs), not only in terms of success rate (≥90% vs ±80%), but even more in terms of duration of normocalcemia (2–4 weeks vs 1–2 weeks). The newer bisphosphonate ibandronate at doses of 2–4 mg can correct TIH in at least 75% of the cases.

Bone Pain

It has not been convincingly demonstrated that currently available oral bisphosphonates can reduce metastatic bone pain. When pooling the available data of several phase II trials with iterative pamidronate infusions, a clear-cut relief of bone pain appeared to occur in more than one third of the cases. Placebo-controlled studies have shown that clodronate and pamidronate infusions can indeed exert significant analgesic effects. With high doses of pamidronate (90–120 mg), a significant analgesic effect is observed in about two thirds of the patients.

Sclerosis of Lytic Bone Lesions

Repeated pamidronate infusions can induce an objective sclerosis of lytic lesions in one-fourth to one-third of the patients. Bisphosphonates can thus lead to bone "recalcification" by themselves and this phenomenon of "recalcification" appears to be similar to what can be achieved by conventional hormone- or chemotherapy. Similarly, an increase in the objective bone response rate to chemotherapy has been shown in a large randomized clinical trial when patients were receiving chemotherapy plus pamidronate as compared to chemotherapy alone, 33% vs 18%, respectively.

The dose of 90 mg of pamidronate appears to be the most adequate to treat the complications of TIO and, based on clinical and biochemical data, infusions should be administered every 3–4 weeks.

Bisphosphonates for the Prevention of Complications of Breast Cancer and Myeloma-induced Osteolysis

Breast Cancer

The low absorption of oral bisphosphonates constitutes a major obstacle to their use as oral drugs in cancer patients. Two large-scale studies in patients with breast cancer metastatic to the skeleton, one with clodronate and one with pamidronate, nevertheless indicate that the prolonged administration of oral bisphosphonates can significantly reduce the frequency of morbid skeletal events, notably the incidence of hypercalcemic episodes, of vertebral deformities and of episodes of severe bone pain. However, they exert no significant effects on the skeletal event-free period, on survival, or on the radiological aspect of lytic lesions and there is only a mild decrease in the need for systemic treatment changes and for radiotherapy on bone lesions. The active daily dose of clodronate is at least 1600 mg/day but a dose-response effect beyond that dose is unknown.

The results obtained with intravenous bisphosphonates are more impressive than with oral compounds. Large scale double-blind randomized placebo-controlled trials comparing monthly 90-mg pamidronate infusions to placebo infusions for one year in addition to chemo- or hormonetherapy in breast cancer patients with at least one lytic bone metastasis have just been completed. The results are particularly impressive in the chemotherapy trial where the median time to the occurrence of the first skeletal-related event was increased by 47% in the pamidronate group (13.1 vs 7.0 months). There was also a significant reduction in the proportion of patients having any skeletal-related event, in the number of non-vertebral pathological fractures, and in the proportion of patients having radiation to bone or surgery on bone, by about one half for each. The objective response rate of bone lesions to chemotherapy was also increased. The follow-up of this trial has shown that the mean skeletal morbidity rate (number of skeletal-related events per year) has been 2.1 in the pamidronate group compared to 3.3 in the placebo group. Placebo-controlled trials with the newer bisphosphonate ibandronate, given orally or intravenously, are ongoing.

Despite the higher efficacy of intravenous bisphosphonates compared to oral compounds, the choice between both routes of administration is influenced by individual circumstances. For example, the intravenous route will be preferred by most clinicians if the patient is already receiving chemotherapy every 3–4 weeks, while the oral route may be preferred for patients receiving hormone therapy. More importantly, the optimal selection of patients for treatment remains to be defined, although it is likely that patients with multiple lytic bone lesions will benefit most. The optimal duration of treatment is also unknown, especially that the criteria for stopping their administration must be different from those used to stop directly antineoplastic drugs. Bisphosphonates are aimed at reducing the complications of bone metastases and they should not necessarily be stopped when metastatic bone disease is evolutive. However, criteria are lacking to determine if and how long a patient benefits from bisphosphonate administration. New biochemical markers of bone resorption may help to identify those patients continuing to benefit from therapy, as preliminary data suggest that a normalization of their concentrations is necessary to have beneficial effects.

Multiple Myeloma

Multiple myeloma is typically characterized by a marked increase in osteoclast activity and proliferation, a phenomenon which could by itself play a contributory role to the growth of myeloma cells in bone. Bisphosphonates appear to be of great benefit for these patients. Clodronate given at 2400 mg daily for two years has been shown to significantly reduce the proportion of patients who develop a progression of lytic bone lesions. Clodronate appears to be effective only in patients who respond to standard chemotherapy, although the benefits become more apparent when the effects of chemotherapy wear off.

The efficacy of regular 90-mg pamidronate infusions in addition to antimyeloma chemotherapy regimen has also been demonstrated in a large scale double-blind placebo-controlled trial. The proportion of patients developing a skeletal-related event was significantly smaller in the pamidronate than in the placebo group, 24% vs 41%, and the mean morbidity rate was 2.1 in the placebo group vs 1.1 in the pamidronate group. Preliminary follow-up data on this trial suggest a prolongation of the survival in the pamidronate group in the patients receiving second or subsequent lines of chemotherapy. These trials indicate that bisphosphonates in addition to chemotherapy are superior to chemotherapy alone in patients with multiple myeloma with lytic lesions, although the optimal duration and doses of treatment are unknown.

Summary

The propensity of breast cancer cells to metastasize in bone could notably be due to the rich supply of relevant growth factors present in the skeletal microenvironment, which could increase breast cancer cell growth. Bone destruction is essentially mediated by osteoclast activation. Bisphosphonates are potent inhibitors of osteoclast-mediated bone resorption that have opened the way for a noncytotoxic treatment of bone metastases. They have become the standard treatment for treating tumor-induced hypercalcemia and, at adequate dose levels (90 mg), the efficacy of pamidronate is not significantly influenced by the tumor type or the degree of metastatic bone involvement. Regular pamidronate infusions can also relieve bone pain probably in more than one third of the cases and an objective sclerosis of osteolytic lesions can be seen in one fourth of the patients. A dose of 90 mg of pamidronate administered every 3–4 weeks could constitute an adequate therapeutic scheme for the treatment of established tumor-induced osteolysis. On the other hand, the prolonged administration of oral bisphosphonates can reduce the frequency of morbid skeletal events by about one fourth. Regular pamidronate infusions have larger effects and they also reduce the proportion of patients having radiation to bone or surgery on bone by about one half. The objective response rate of bone lesions to chemotherapy is also increased. On the other hand, regular pamidronate infusions in addition to antimyeloma chemotherapy regimen in myeloma patients can reduce the mean morbidity rate by almost 50%. Lastly, therapy with bisphosphonates also has the advantage to prevent postmenopausal osteoporosis in women cured from breast cancer for whom estrogen replacement therapy is still considered to be contraindicated.

Suggested Reading

Body JJ, Coleman RE, Piccart M. (1996) Use of bisphosphonates in cancer patients. *Cancer Treat Rev* 22: 265–287.

Hortobagyi GN, Theriault RL, Porter L et al. (1996) Efficacy of pamidronate in reducing skeletal complications in patients with breast cancer and lytic bone metastases. *N Engl J Med* 335: 1785–1791.

Fleisch H. (1997) *Bisphosphonates in Bone Disease – From the Laboratory to the Patient*, 3rd edn. The Parthenon Publishing Group, Carnforth

25

Osteoporosis During Young Adulthood

Robert Marcus

Investigators in the bone field have long considered osteoporosis to be exclusively a condition of bone loss. We understand now that successful acquisition of bone during adolescence is a major determinant of final adult bone mass and powerfully affects later bone loss and fragility. Indeed, the variance around values for peak bone mass far exceeds the amount of bone that is lost during later adult life. Adolescence represents a period of opportunity when appropriate attention to lifestyle factors, particularly diet and physical activity, permit optimal development of a bone mass commensurate with that programmed by genetic endowment. Failure to attend to these factors may lead to diminished peak bone mass and a higher risk for subsequent fracture.

Genetic Influences on Bone Acquisition

About 75% of the variance in peak bone mineral density (BMD) is genetically determined, and considerable interest has centered about identifying the specific responsible genes. The BMD measurement itself is highly influenced by bone size, so these genes include those that determine body size, such as genes related to the Growth Hormone/Insulin-like Growth Factor-I axis. A major role in skeletal development has been shown for estrogen in both boys and girls, and a polymorphism in the estradiol receptor also appears to influence bone acquisition. Polymorphisms of the vitamin D receptor gene have been inconsistently associated with bone mass, but little work has been reported to date that relates this polymorphism to bone acquisition.

Environmental Influences on Bone Acquisition

Among the lifestyle factors that could be implicated in successful bone acquisition, dietary calcium and weight-bearing physical activity have the strongest experimental support. Clinical trials consistently show greater bone acquisition when supplemental calcium is given. However, the ultimate impact of supplementation on adult bone mass remains in doubt, since differences between treatment groups dissipate shortly after stopping the supplement. Particularly in teenage girls, average habitual dietary calcium is well-below recommended levels, making dietary calcium a limiting nutrient for bone acquisition in a large segment of the teenage population. Within limits, increased physical activity has been consistently associated with improved bone density throughout growth and development. Sustained immobilization during adolescence may severely jeopardize bone acquisition. In years past, long-term bed rest for a teenager with acute rheumatic carditis is an example of this type of restricted activity.

By contrast, some adolescent girls exercise to the point that menstrual function ceases and circulating estradiol reverts to a prepubertal range. Such girls exhibit substantial deficits in bone mass. Depending on the patient's age, these may represent interruption of bone acquisition, bone loss, or a combination of the two. Athletes most likely to develop exercise associated amenorrhea are those who participate in endurance events, such as long-distance running, and who initiated serious exercise training prior to or within a short interval after menarche. Ballet dancers and gymnasts are also highly susceptible to oligo/amenorrhea. Some evidence indicates that women gymnasts actually show unexpectedly *high* BMD values, perhaps reflecting the high impact nature of their training.

Other lifestyle factors that likely impair bone acquisition in teenage girls include early pregnancy, and ethanol or tobacco use. However, very little specific information has been reported concerning these factors during the growth years.

Specific Examples of Acquisitional Osteopenia

Inherited Disorders

Osteoporosis is a *sine qua non* for inherited mutations in the type I collagen gene, known collectively as Osteogenesis Imperfecta (OI). Some young adults with osteoporosis may have subclinical forms of OI that represent unique and difficult-to-identify mutations in collagen or other bone-specific proteins. Other important genetic disorders also lead to osteoporosis in young adults. Cystic Fibrosis (CF) is associated in adults with profound osteopenia. It is difficult to find any consistent aspect of the disease or its treatment that is related to bone mass. Exposure to corticosteroids, hypogonadism, and intestinal malabsorption are all common but highly individual. Nonetheless, with more successful early therapy, survival into the 3rd and 4th decades and beyond has become common for CF patients, and it is appropriate to pay attention to long-term skeletal health. Appropriate supplementation with calcium and vitamin D, and estrogen or testosterone replacement are clearly indicated. If patients experience fractures, a potent bisphosphonate is likely to offer benefit.

Marfan syndrome is associated with low BMD, primarily in the appendicular skeleton. In addition, the femoral neck length in these patients is significantly increased. The combination of low BMD and long hip axis length makes such patients at uniquely high long-term risk for hip fracture. Just as with CF, Marfan patients now survive well beyond the 4th decade, largely the result of successful surgical repair of the thoracic aorta. Thus, Marfan women should be considered likely candidates for hormone replacement therapy at the time of menopause.

Osteoporosis Due to Environmental Factors

Anything that jeopardizes cyclic reproductive function in women may lead to bone loss. In particular, exercise-associated amenorrhea has been discussed above. Successful treatment requires encouraging the woman to decrease her exercise volume to the point that menses return. Women who remain amenorrheic but are given supplemental calcium and/or estrogen appear not to achieve important gains in bone mass. Frequently, such women have been amenorrheic for several years, and recovery of bone mass in that setting seems to be particularly disappointing.

Anorexia nervosa is a common disorder of young women. It is associated with severe deficits in bone mass. When patients are in their teen years, these deficits mostly reflect failure to acquire bone; later on, bone loss may be the primary mechanism. Although estrogen deficiency may contribute, the most important determinant of bone deficits in anorexia nervosa is the decrease in body weight. Similarly, weight rehabilitation is the most important predictor of improvement in bone mass. Calcium or estrogen alone or in combination are not effective unless weight is also restored toward normal. The use of potent bisphosphonates for patients with these conditions is probably indicated if they are experiencing fracture. However, no published data yet support this approach.

Treatment of Low Bone Mass in Young People

General hygienic interventions, such as dietary or supplemental calcium and adequate physical activity (customized for individual tolerance) are recommended for virtually all patients. Recommendation of drug therapy, however, is problematic. The impact of potent bisphosphonates on bone acquisition is not certain, nor is it clear that young individuals with low bone mass derive sufficient gains in BMD or anti-fracture benefit to justify using these agents prior to the times in life when bone loss begins to be an important factor. For the present, I reserve their use for patients who have, in addition to low BMD, already experienced at least one low-trauma fracture.

26

Immobilization, Exercise and Osteoporosis

Mehrsheed Sinaki

Immobilization and Bone Loss

Bone is exposed to constantly changing patterns of loading and adapts to these changes through alterations in bone mass and skeletal geometry. Decreased weight bearing and immobilization are known stimuli to bone resorption. Weightlessness in space travel has been reported to result in a 33% loss of trabecular bone volume over a 25-week period. There is sufficient evidence to support the concept that the absence of pressure forces on the skeleton is primarily responsible for disuse osteopenia. However, the exact mechanism whereby bone mineral is lost is uncertain. Mechanical strain on the matrix stimulates bone formation at the cellular or molecular level. The mechanism by which the mechanical signal is transduced into a biochemical signal is not known.

The rehabilitative management of osteoporosis consists of; (1) management of established osteoporosis and (2) rehabilitative management of complications.

Established Osteoporosis

The objectives of the rehabilitative program for established osteoporosis are to maintain or improve posture, relieve or lessen pain, increase activity, and improve safety of ambulation. A progressive sound strengthening exercise program for axial and appendicular musculature can decrease the risk of falls. In addition, increasing mobility can reduce concomitant low self-esteem and depression. The feeling of being locked in a fragile skeleton can, at times, be distressing. It may be helpful to consider counseling and psychiatric help for severe depression. If skeletal fragility interferes with antigravity exercises, the progressive rehabilitation program can be initiated with "in-water" exercises.

Skeletal Complications Related to Osteoporosis

Along with the treatment outlined above, the following measures should be considered for complications of osteoporosis; spinal supports and gait assistive devices to improve patient's posture, prevent falls, restore confidence, increase activity, and improve balance. Maintenance of musculoskeletal flexibility and coordination will allow the patient freedom to participate in weight-bearing and loading exercises. Implementation of sedative physiotherapy such as application of cold at the acute stage and moist heat and mild stroking massage at the chronic stage can decrease muscular pain and related malposture.

Mechanical loading whether related to healthy body weight or weight training exercises contributes to skeletal health. Weight-bearing exercises such as walking and stair climbing can decrease age-related bone loss. However, discontinuation of these activities results in a reduction of bone mass to baseline levels. Upper extremity loading exercises expose the vertebral bodies to compressive forces that can be beyond the biomechanical competence of the osteoporotic spine. Therefore, they should be limited and used with proper techniques. Improvement of back extensor strength can reduce kyphotic posture and risk of vertebral fracture. Back exercises should consist of a combination of back extension and isometric lumbar flexion exercises to avoid increased sacral inclination (Figure 26.1).

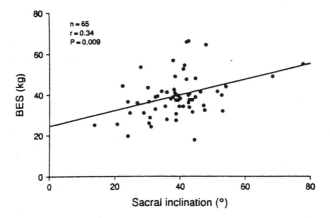

Figure 26.1. Significant positive correlation between back extensor strength and sacral inclination in 65 healthy, active, estrogen-deficient women aged 48–65 years. From Sinaki et al; *Am J Phys Med Rehabil* 75(5); 370–374, 1996 (by permission).

Back Supports

Back supports are used in an attempt to support and correct posture as much as possible. Semirigid or rigid back supports are used, depending on the severity of the spinal osteoporosis, the patient's tolerance, and the acuity of compression fracture.

In cases of acute compression fracture, the purpose of supporting the spine is to expedite ambulation while allowing rest for the painful area of the back. Patients can be instructed to perform isometric exercises while wearing their back support. Supports used for pain sometimes have to be applied for a prolonged period, in which case atrophy of the back muscles may result. Physiotherapy is necessary to prevent this atrophy and should include exercises that strengthen the trunk muscles and provide muscular stability (Figure 26.2).

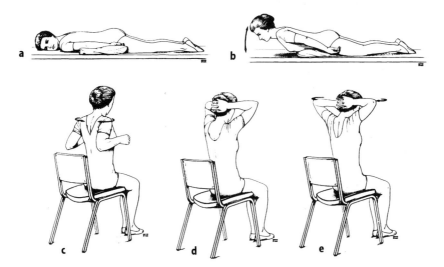

Figure 26.2. (a)-(c) Back extension exercises; (a), (b) In prone position, (c) In sitting position. This position avoids or minimizes pain in patients with severe osteoporosis. (d), (e) Deep-breathing exercise combined with pectoral stretching and back extension exercise. Patient sits on a chair, locks her hands behind her head, and inhales deeply while she gently extends her elbows backward. While exhaling, she returns to the starting position. This is repeated 10 to 15 times. Figures (b), (c), and (e) modified from Sinaki (1982) *Mayo Clin Proc* 57:699–703 with permission; Figures (a) and (d) from Sinaki (1995) In: Riggs BL, Melton LJ III (eds) *Osteoporosis; Etiology, Diagnosis and Management,* 2nd edn. Lippincott-Raven Publishers, Philadelphia Chapter 20, pp 435–473, with permission.

Exposure of the fragile skeleton to physical exertion beyond its biomechanical competence during activities of daily living or recreational activities can be deleterious. Avoidance of strenuous physical activities is recommended. An exercise program for the fragile skeleton needs to be progressive with supervision in the early stages. Avoidance of kyphotic posturing through use of a weighted kypho-orthosis (Posture Training Support or PTS) and a daily exercise program is highly recommended. The PTS can be used in patients with a lack of tolerance for other spinal supports or in patients who have kyphotic posturing despite thoracolumbar supports. The PTS can also be used as a method of educational biofeedback and proprioceptive training for prevention of kyphotic posturing of the osteoporotic spine during activities of daily living. PTS can also improve ambulatory posture and decrease the tendency to fall in patients who develop axial instability with aging or other degenerative central nervous system disorders.

Cardiovascular Conditioning and Fragile Skeleton

Immobility is associated with loss of muscle strength, loss of BMD and reduction of cardiovascular fitness. Exercises that are beneficial for fitness and cardiovascular conditioning are not necessarily weight-bearing and effective for improvement of bone mineral density. Not all types of exercises are safe for the osteoporotic spine. In severe osteoporosis, if improvement of cardiovascular condition is indicated, swimming or simply walking in water can be a good, safe start. Immobile patients may also benefit from water exercises before starting antigravity exercises.

The effect of immobility when added to the presence of connective tissue diseases exacerbates bone loss. The combination of collagen disease and immobility in rheumatoid arthritis results in a significant reduction of bone mass, especially at the proximal femur. Indeed, the fracture risk is increased by about 100% in rheumatoid arthritis patients. These patients will benefit from regular daily isometric muscle contraction exercises which can help to preserve muscles despite the inflammation of the joints. Patients who suffer a period of immobility in bed need to resume their daily activities plus some additional exertional exercises with supervision.

Implementing exercise programs which include safe ambulatory activities with use of gait assistive devices can improve skeletal loading which is so needed.

Assistive Devices

The use of assistive devices (canes or walkers) is of utmost importance to improve safety during patient's ambulatory activities.

Gait-assistive devices include a conventional cane, supportive canes with a broader base of support and prongs, walkers, and wheeled walkers. Walkers are more supportive than canes and are used for limited ambulatory activities. In cases of prolonged immobility, the ambulatory activities can be initiated with sitting position and use of a wheelchair with progression to standing and use of gait aids. As the patient's improvement allows, weight-bearing and weight-training programs can also be initiated.

In addition to the above rehabilitative measures, other factors such as nutrition and pharmacological intervention must be considered. A daily calcium intake of 1500 mg and daily vitamin D intake of 600 to 800 IU is recommended. The detrimental effect of postmenopausal bone loss can be reduced with proper pharmacological intervention including hormone replacement therapy, use of calcitonin, or alendronate sodium. These measures will be discussed in other chapters.

Suggested Reading

American College of Rheumatology Task Force on Osteoporosis Guidelines. (1996) Recommendations for the Prevention and Treatment of Glucocorticoid-Induced Osteoporosis. *Arth and Rheum* 39(11): 1791–1801.

Folz TJ, Sinaki M. (1995) A nouveau aid for posture training in degenerative disorders of the central nervous system. *J of Musculoskeletal Pain* 3(4): 59–69.

Lynn S, Sinaki M, Westerlind K. (1997) Balance characteristics of individuals with osteoporosis. *Arch Phys Med Rehabil* 78(3): 273–277.

Rodan GA. (1991) Mechanical loading, estrogen deficiency, and the coupling of bone formation to bone resorption [review]. *J Bone Miner Res* 6(6): 527–530.

Sinaki M. (1993) Metabolic bone disease. In: Sinaki M (ed) *Basic Clinical Rehabilitation Medicine*, 2nd edn. Mosby Year Book Inc., Chicago, pp. 209–236.

Sinaki M. (1995) Musculoskeletal management. In: Riggs BL, Melton LJ III (eds) *Osteoporosis; Etiology, Diagnosis and Management*, 2nd edn. Lippincott-Raven Publishers, Philadelphia, pp 435–473.

Sinaki M. (1996) The effect of physical activity on bone: A review. *Current Opinion in Rheumatology* 8(4): 376–383.

Sinaki M, Itoi E, Rogers J, Bergstralh E, Wahner H (1996) Relationship of posture to bone density, back strength, and physical activity in postmenopausal women. *Am J Phys Med and Rehabil* 75(5): 370–374.

Sinaki M, Wollan P, Scott R, Gelczer R. (1996) Can strong back extensors prevent vertebral fractures in women with osteoporosis? *Mayo Clin Proc* 71(10): 951–956.

27

Nutrition and Osteoporosis

Peter Burckhardt

The impact of nutrition on bone varies over the main periods of life (growth and adolescence, mature adulthood, early postmenopause, senescence) in its nature and in its importance. Nutrition influences growth and development of peak bone mass and maintenance of adult bone mass, modifies postmenopausal bone loss, and has an important impact on bone loss and bone health in advanced age. Although mainly considered as an environmental factor, nutrition, respectively its impact on bone, is influenced by genetic conditions. For example, the effect of a calcium supplementation in calcium deficiency depends partially on the vitamin D-receptor gene allele. Despite this, and despite the fact that nutrition accounts maximally for 20% of the variance of peak bone mass, it represents a modifiable factor in the pathogenesis of osteoporosis offering the possibility for corrective interventions.

The major nutritional components of which the influence on bone has been studied, are the following: calcium, vitamin D, protein and sodium.

Calcium

Intake, Absorption, Losses

Calcium intake varies geographically, but is not correlated with the geographic incidence of osteoporosis. It is low (300–600 mg per day) in some Asiatic countries, higher in the US and highest in Northern Europe (average about 1400 mg in some countries). It mostly depends on habits acquired during childhood, and decreases in senescence.

The need for growth (girls ± 145, boys ± 185 mg/day) should be covered by the nutritional intake. In addition, the obligatory losses should be compensated at all ages, including those by urine, feces and the skin. They sum up to an average of 300 mg, minimum 150 mg. They are probably smaller when calcium intake is constantly low, due to adaptive mechanisms, but they cannot be measured individually on a routine basis.

Calcium absorption efficiency depends on age and intake: in postmenopausal women, it is between 20 and 25% at an intake of 1 g, and 30% at an intake of 0.5 g. Absorption lowers with age, together with a loss of adaptation to a low intake. Absorption is enhanced when calcium is given together with food and in several doses.

About 50–70% of dietary calcium comes by dairy products. Sardines, nuts and some vegetables (broccoli) are less important, although relatively rich in calcium, because consumed in smaller amounts. Calcium from milk, cheese, yogurt and from mineral water, is as well absorbed as calcium from commercially available supplements. Reported differences between various preparations are clinically irrelevant for normal gastric pH.

The administration of 1 g of calcium or more decreases PTH secretion, bone resorption and $1,25(OH)_2$ vitamin D_3 levels. Because absorption is enhanced when calcium is given with food and in several daily doses, calcium should be prescribed at doses of maximum 500 mg at once and not in the fasting state The nocturnal rise of bone resorption cannot be decreased by calcium given in the evening or at bed time, since it is caused by the physical inactivity of the night rest. Therefore, calcium should be prescribed with the meals, at any time.

Recommended Intakes

Since obligatory losses can not be determined for a given individual, they should be estimated at 300 mg. Assuming an absorption of 20–25%, an intake of 1200–1500 mg would be necessary for maintaining an equilibrated calcium balance.

The Effect on Bone

Childhood and Adolescence

Optimal nutrition is necessary for the full development of the genetic potential. High calcium intake correlates with higher bone mass in school children, in puberty and in adolescence, although it is not certain that this effect persists. Supplementation with dairy products seems to cause longer lasting effects than with calcium salts. Premenopausal women remembering regular milk intake at childhood have higher lumbar BMD. In any case, malnutrition and anorexia lead to osteoporosis, and insufficient calcium intake probably to suboptimal peak bone mass. All this justifies the recommendation of an adequate calcium intake, if possible in form of dairy products, during growth and adolescence.

Adulthood and Premenopause

Calcium favors the maintenance of BMD together with physical activity, but its effect on premenopausal bone loss is uncertain. Therefore, an adequate nutritional calcium intake is recommended for premenopausal women, but it is unnecessary to prescribe a calcium supplementation unless there is a high risk of osteoporosis or a distinctively low calcium intake.

Early Postmenopause

Bone loss in this period does not depend from calcium intake, but from the lack of estrogens. For this reason, calcium supplementation usually has no significant effect during the first years after menopause. Nevertheless high calcium intake was associated with higher BMD before and after the menopause; but it does not influence the amount of bone loss in-between.

Late Menopause

Calcium supplementation inhibits bone loss, if intake is low. It acts mostly on cortical bone, but a positive effect on lumbar BMD has also been reported with 2 g of calcium, decreasing bone loss without preventing it. The effect of calcium supplementation is reinforced in postmenopausal, elderly women, when combined with exercise.

Senescence

Over the age of 70 years, calcium intake correlates with bone density, when the initial intake is below 900 mg. Calcium supplementation at this age decreases bone loss almost by half, and over 80 years even by 2 to 4% per year. In elderly women, calcium intake is correlated with BMD at all hip sites, especially at the femoral neck. It therefore seems that with increasing age, calcium supplementation is of growing importance, because normal intake declines and absorptive adaptation to low intake disappears.

Influence on Fracture Incidence

Calcium intake correlates with fracture risk, when intake is very low, but not necessarily when intake is high. Therefore calcium intake must be sufficient, i.e. 1200–1500 mg per day, but not very high. When intake is low, calcium supplementation decreases hip fracture risk in postmenopausal women and also the risk of vertebral fractures. It has also been clearly demonstrated that high calcium intake with food or with supplements, decreases hip fracture incidence in elderly persons.

Calcium in the Treatment of Osteoporosis

Given to osteoporotics, calcium decreases bone resorption, increases slightly BMD or decreases bone loss. Hip fracture rate can be decreased when the initial calcium intake was low. The same applies to vertebral fractures in elderly women. But no effect of calcium was yet observed in women without vertebral fractures. As an adjuvant to medical treatment of osteoporosis, calcium is added to all treatments of osteoporosis (bisphosphonates, calcitonin, fluoride, estrogens, etc.). In antiresorptive treatments, it helps to avoid hypocalcemic reactions and inappropriate stimulation of PTH, and in the treatment with fluoride it avoids mineralization defects. In all events, it covers the need for a positivation of bone balance.

Vitamin D

Source, Intake, Requirements

Vitamin D is produced in the skin (UV irradiation), and supplied by food, especially fish and dairy products. In parts of the US, 40% of young adults and a large proportion of elderly women are vitamin D deficient, at least in winter. Up to 60% of elderly persons and the majority of residents of homes for elderlies, as well as chronically hospitalized patients are vitamin D deficient. They are confined to indoor life and therefore depend from vitamin D intake from food. However, their intake is inadequate, in homes only of 50–150 IU per day. When plasma levels drop below 25–30 nmol/l, PTH levels rise, and at even lower levels, also alkaline phosphatase rises. This secondary hyperparathyroidism indicates increased bone turnover, in addition to eventual insufficient mineralization. This occurs mainly in the elderly, residents of homes, but also in postmenopausal women, when the vitamin D intake and sun exposure provide less than 200 IU per day.

Effect on Bone and Recommendations

Low plasma levels of 25OH-Vitamin D_3 correlate also with decreased vertebral BMD, especially in elderlies. Below 30 nmol/l, they correlate with decreasing BMD at the proximal femur. On the other side, elderlies with relatively high vitamin D levels have significantly higher femoral BMD, but equal lumbar or radial BMD. Therefore, vitamin D deficiency seems to have an almost specific effect on the cortical bone on the femoral neck. Indeed, women with hip fractures show lower 25OH-Vitamin D_3 levels, and elderly people with low vitamin D and elevated PTH levels show an accelerated bone loss and an elevated risk for hip fracture.

Recommendations

Elderly persons living in homes and with an intake of only 150 IU should be supplemented by at least 400 IU, which is the minimal required dose in the case of a low calcium intake. Considering that elderly persons take only about 20 IU when they do not drink milk, and 30 to 150 IU with milk, substitution with 400 IU would bring the total intake up to 500 IU.

Vitamin D supplements of 400 to 800 IU per day normalize the 25OH-Vitamin D_3 and PTH levels. In addition, the treatment increases lumbar BMD, and femoral BMD slightly, as long as the calcium intake is low.

But 400 IU could not prevent hip fracture and the same dose given to postmenopausal women decreased bone loss only when calcium was added. 800 IU given to postmenopausal women, in the average over 60 years, decreased femoral bone loss by half, but did not influence vertebral BMD. It needed 800 IU given together with 1 or 1.2 g of calcium in order to decrease hip fracture incidence in the elderly by almost 50%. Therefore, vitamin D supplementation is important for the femoral neck already in the 60's, and significantly decreases hip fracture incidence in elderlies.

The effect of vitamin D is the same when the supplement is given as an intermittent high dose or as a daily low dose. It is almost impossible to replace the lack of vitamin D due to the absence of direct sun light by vitamin D from dietary sources. Enrichment of milk with vitamin D or of margarine, or even bread, as done in certain countries, does not guarantee a sufficient intake. Only regular consumption of fish (not deep frozen, not smoked) would provide enough, but for most countries, this is either unusual or too expensive. For this reason, supplementation by vitamin D is recommended in elderly osteoporotics, and for prevention of osteoporosis in all elderly persons living indoors.

Proteins

Sufficient protein intake is essential for bone health. Protein malnutrition during childhood and adolescence leads to growth retardation and to low peak bone mass, the extreme example being anorexia nervosa. The positive effect of proteins is partially explained by its stimulatory effect on the secretion of the insulin-like growth factor (IGF). During adulthood and senescence, the needs for proteins are constant, but intake declines with age. Low protein intake in elderlies, a frequent phenomenon, contributes to bone loss. Protein supplementation in elderlies increases femoral BMD.

Excessive protein intake was associated with a higher risk for osteoporosis and osteoporotic fractures. This might apply to animal protein (meat), but not to vegetal proteins such as soya. Indeed, the metabolism of dietary animal proteins produces organic acids, respectively acid residues, which need to be buffered and eliminated. They contribute to a trend to a metabolic acidosis which increases urinary calcium excretion. On the other hand, bone being the main source of buffers (mainly carbonate), metabolic acidosis stimulates the release of calcium from bone by chemical effects and by stimulation of osteoclasts, and also inhibits osteoblast function. This might explain why a constant high intake of dietary animal proteins can lead to a negative calcium balance and to increased bone loss. It remains open, if vegetal proteins have a more positive long term effect on bone. But despite this potential negative effect of a high intake of animal protein, protein deficiency must be strictly avoided.

Sodium

Intake of salt has largely increased over the last 200 years, especially in non maritime regions. High sodium intake increases urinary calcium excretion and contributes to a negative calcium balance. By varying sodium intake, not only calcium excretion can be modulated, but also that of markers of bone resorption. It is possible that this effect depends more on the anion chloride, than on sodium. Although it is probable that the secular increase of salt intake over some generations contributed to the secular increase of osteoporosis, epidemiologic data proving this are lacking. The same applies to the long term effect to the potentially calcium sparing effect of salt restriction. In case of hypercalciuria, it is however recommended to reduce an eventually high intake of salt as the first therapeutic intervention.

Other Nutritional Factors

Vitamin K stimulates bone formation, partially because it is essential for gammacarboxylation of osteocalcin. Low vitamin K levels correlate with low BMD, with lower osteocalcin and with increased hip fracture risk. But vitamin K deficiency is not an isolated cause of osteoporosis, since it is usually part of clinically more alarming conditions such as e.g. malabsorption. If vitamin K insufficiency contributes as a co-factor to osteoporosis in the elderly, remains an open question, since its diagnosis depends on costly measurements.

The influence of various trace minerals such as zinc, selenium, strontium on bone health is still poorly documented. It is still possible, that chronic insufficiency in these trace elements is frequent and exerts a chronic negative effect on bone, but prospective and interventional studies are scarce.

Mineral Waters

Mineral waters are recognized as a natural source of calcium. In certain cases, they contain almost half as much calcium as milk. Calcium from mineral water is as well absorbed as that from dairy products. However, it would be wrong to consider mineral water as an only source of calcium. First, it contains a variable amount of sodium, which might increase urinary calcium losses. Finally, it contains a variable amount of bicarbonate. High intake of bicarbonate decreases bone resorption, decreases urinary calcium excretion and stimulates bone formation. By that it has a positive effect on calcium balance. It is therefore probable, that the content of bicarbonate in mineral water is at least as important as that of calcium.

28

The Menopause: A Woman's View

Rosemary Rowe & Linda Edwards

Question a group of women about their attitude towards the menopause and the replies you receive will be highly diverse. Some will subscribe to the male conspiracy theory that doctors have over-medicalized the problem in order to extend their power over women and that "the change" is purely a natural event in one's life. Others will regard it as a major point of transition in a woman's life sometimes viewed negatively as the beginning of old age, sometimes viewed positively as a time when women enjoy greater freedom. A small minority may recognize that it is a time when women become estrogen deficient, a state which needs to be carefully managed to avoid long-term problems such as osteoporosis or heart disease.

For health care professionals this bewildering range of responses may be enough to dissuade them from even tackling the issue. How can general protocols be effective when confronted by such a range of attitudes which will strongly influence willingness to accept medical advice let alone commence and continue with therapeutic agents? In these cost conscious days, the whole process is likely to be so time consuming that many healthcare professionals may balk at investing resources into an exercise with no guaranteed successful outcome. However such a nihilist approach cannot be justified when the cost of non-intervention in terms of morbidity and mortality from osteoporosis and cardiovascular disease is so high.

Most women will live a third of their lives post menopause and healthcare professionals have a responsibility for enabling their patients to enjoy as high a quality of life as possible during this time. To achieve this goal it is vital that doctors and other medical staff understand what influences a woman's attitude to the menopause, what concerns they have regarding prophylactic interventions and how they can in turn encourage women to take appropriate steps to maintain their long-term health and well-being.

Surveys have shown that whilst women identify health care professionals as an important source of information regarding the menopause many do not consult their doctor at this time, relying on information gleaned from alternative sources including friends, family and the media which may vary considerably in the reliability of the information and advice offered. These different information sources together with the individual woman's personal experience of menopause will shape her attitude towards it. If a woman's experience of menopause is positive and generally problem free she may regard it with relief as a liberation from premenstrual syndrome (PMS), period pains and monthly bleeding. In such circumstances she is unlikely to request support from her general practitioner and may thereby fail to receive advice and information on long term health issues that arise as a result of estrogen deficiency. If a woman is both socially and economically disadvantaged she is unlikely to find the time to "bother" her doctor about menopausal symptoms and just simply put up with them, as her mother did.

In contrast, female health care professionals and women who are regularly exposed to medical professionals, such as the wives of gynaecologists, are more likely to seek advice and follow recommendations for treatment (see reference attached). Social and cultural factors are therefore just as likely as physical symptoms to influence women's attitudes to the menopause and whether they are willing to seek medical advice.

Whether a woman is receptive to advice given will depend partly on her attitude to the menopause and partly on concerns she may have regarding treatment, and in particular hormone replacement therapy (HRT). For those women who regard the menopause as just a "natural event" with which we should not interfere, there is often great resistance to take hormones. This, together with anxiety regarding the possible increased risk of breast cancer, fears of alleged weight gain with HRT and a reluctance to continue or resume monthly bleeding, explains the very low uptake of HRT. A woman's views will also be shaped by the experience of her friends and family. If female friends have suffered side effects such as bloating and breast tenderness from HRT and have discontinued therapy she will be much less willing to try HRT for herself. However, if her mother suffered from osteoporosis there is evidence now that this will persuade her to take HRT. Similarly if there is a history of breast cancer in the family it is highly unlikely that HRT will be considered an option. The physician's response to menopause queries will also influence future behavior. A lukewarm or negative response to a request for advice on HRT, — perhaps an overemphasis of the risks of breast cancer after 5–10 years on therapy, and the patient is likely to seek a further consultation.

Attitudes are further confused for those women who experience an early menopause, before age 45, either naturally or surgically induced. Many women find symptoms of approaching menopause at this age, as ovaries begin to fail, all the more distressing if their doctor dismisses them without investigation as being "too young". Some find themselves battling with no diagnosis or inappropriate prescriptions for anti-depressants which further confuses the issues.

Given all these different factors that influence a woman's attitude and response to menopause, how can healthcare professionals provide appropriate support and advice? The first step is to be conscious of the different health beliefs and concerns that women hold and to develop services which recognize this diversity. Waiting for women to present in the surgery may not be appropriate, as those who need advice most may well not wish to "bother" their GP. Some mechanism is required to ensure that all women approaching the menopause receive information and advice — especially those with premature ovarian failure. This may be through group meetings held in the evening, well woman clinics, or may be through group meetings held in the evening, well woman clinics, or opportunistic advice offered at the time that a woman attends for a cervical smear, or individual consultations.

One-off advice is unlikely to answer all her questions so it is sensible to establish a two stage procedure which involves the woman seeing the practice nurse first for general advice and information about the menopause followed by time for her to consider this information and then an appointment with the GP at which she can raise any outstanding concerns. All discussions need to include a review of the individual's personal and family history as well as consideration of the various treatment options available. Involvement in the decisionmaking process is critical for women to have a realistic understanding of the likely benefits of taking HRT and for them to feel sufficiently committed to persist with therapy in spite of initial side effects. Recall is vitally important to ensure that women are taking treatments prescribed and to ensure that short term side effects are monitored and alternative therapies prescribed if side effects continue to be troublesome.

Women's physiological and psychological response to the menopause varies enormously. Providing good information and advice and opportunities for women to express their concerns are vitally important if physicians are to assist women in coping with both its short and long-term effects. Patient societies such as the National Osteoporosis Society (in the U.K.) offer valuable assistance to healthcare professionals by providing well balanced patient literature, resources for medical staff and in encouraging the media to portray a balanced view of the menopause. It is only through this partnership of care that women and their physicians will feel empowered to adopt a positive approach to the menopause and its long-term consequences.

Suggested Reading

Greer G. (1991) *The Change: Women, Ageing and the Menopause*. Hamish Hamilton, London.

Hope S, Rees CMP. (1995) Why British women start and stop hormone replacement therapy. *J Br Meno Soc* 1(2): 26–28.

Isaacs AJ, Britton AR, McPherson K. (1995) Utilisation of hormone replacement therapy by women doctors. *BMJ* 311: 1399–1401.

Roberts PJ. (1991) The menopause and hormone replacement therapy: views of women in general practice receiving hormone replacement therapy. *Br J Gen Prac* 41: 421–424.

Brockie J. (1996) Role of the nurse in patient compliance with HRT. *J Br Meno Soc* 2: 19–21.

Draper J, Roland M. (1990) Perimenopausal women's views on taking hormone replacement therapy to prevent osteoporosis. *BMJ* 300: 786–788.

29

Future Developments: Risk Assessment

Philip D. Ross

While there are many risk factors for fractures among the elderly, this discussion is restricted to assessment using risk factors related to osteoporosis — that is, those related to bone strength.

Radiographic Absorptiometry

One of the earliest techniques for measuring bone densitometry is radiographic absorptiometry (RA), which quantitates bone mineral density (BMD) by comparing the bone image density on a standard radiograph to a reference range, usually based on an aluminum wedge included in the exposure field. The traditional RA approach was temporarily abandoned when newer techniques such as photon and x-ray absorptiometry were developed, partly because of problems with precision. However, computerized analysis has improved the precision considerably, and the RA technique is currently enjoying a revival. Two common measurement sites are the finger (phalanges) and hand (metacarpal). The precision is approximately 1% for the phalanges measurement, and 2% for the metacarpal. Both measurements predict fracture risk as well as other BMD measurements.

A new RA approach has been developed which acquires and calculates BMD in a single step using a dedicated table-top unit to perform film-less imaging, thereby eliminating the need for expensive standard radiography equipment, as well as the additional time and cost of developing and analyzing images on film. While RA appears to be perfectly suitable for screening and assessing fracture risk, its role in monitoring treatment is less certain, because there is some evidence that changes in phalanges BMD during treatment may not be as large as those seen at other sites such as the spine. However, other techniques have shortcomings as well; spine BMD measurements are often adversely affected by osteo-arthritis and other conditions. The usefulness of RA and other measures for monitoring changes over time should become clear in the near future as more longitudinal data emerge.

Quantitative Ultrasound

Quantitative ultrasound (QUS) measurements measure the propagation of non-ionizing ultrasound waves to evaluate characteristics of bone related to strength and elasticity. It is not certain what bone characteristics QUS actually measures, and changes in QUS during treatment may or may not accurately reflect changes in bone strength (the same may be true of BMD to some extent). QUS measurements are often performed at the calcaneus because it contains a large proportion of trabecular bone, but measurements at other sites (such as the tibia, patella, and phalanges) have also been developed. Heel QUS measurements are similar to BMD measurements in their ability to predict fractures. Furthermore, QUS may complement BMD by providing additional information about bone strength. Thus, QUS promises to be an important modality for assessing fracture risk, especially considering the portability, speed, and lack of ionizing radiation. Although the radiation exposure associated with standard BMD measurements is much lower than natural radiation exposure levels, patient perceptions may sometimes favor the use of QUS, as in measurements of children. QUS may also have economic and logistic advantages in communities which restrict the use of x-ray densitometry.

Bone Geometry and Structure

Hip axis length (HAL) and other measures of bone geometry are associated with hip fracture risk. Although such measurements may help to identify which patients are at high risk of fractures, it is unlikely that treatment will modify HAL; therefore, BMD (or possibly QUS or biochemical markers) must be relied on to monitor the effectiveness of treatment. If hip BMD is measured, HAL represents additional, "free" information that can be used to complement BMD for assessing fracture risk. However, if other BMD measurements are obtained routinely instead of hip BMD, then obtaining HAL incurs additional costs.

Fractal analysis and other image analysis techniques are being developed to provide information about bone structure (micro-architecture) to complement BMD for evaluating bone strength and fracture risk using standard radiographs, magnetic resonance imaging, or computed tomography. Analysis of regional differences in BMD within single bones such as the hip or vertebral body is also a promising technique, but may be limited to assessing risk at specific fracture sites (such as the hip) rather than general fracture risk. Morphometric imaging of the spine has also been developed for diagnosing vertebral fractures; this technique may have advantages over conventional radiography because the x-ray beam remains perpendicular to the spine at all levels. However, poor resolution in the upper spine remains a problem at present.

The Future of Risk Assessment

By its very definition, prevention requires that intervention begins prior to the occurrence of fractures. To accomplish this without needlessly treating people with low risk, screening to identify high risk individuals will be necessary. Thus, all women should be evaluated at the time of menopause, as well as elderly men and people of any age with major risk factors such as hypogonadism or corticosteroid use.

Inexpensive, compact methods such as appendicular densitometry (including RA) and QUS will largely replace DXA for widespread screening. Mass production and technical refinements can reduce the cost to the point where skeletal risk assessment will be accessible in most physicians' offices. Given safety, speed, convenience, and low cost, screening of children and adolescents will probably become common, enabling skeletal deficiencies to be identified and corrected during development, thereby reducing the need for treatment later in life. The general practitioner will almost certainly play a key role in evaluating skeletal development in children and fracture risk in adults, because there are no symptoms or other tell-tale signs of osteoporosis and osteopenia.

Interpretation

Fracture risk exists along a continuum which is much larger in range than is apparent from simply using a single cutoff (such as a T-score < -2.5). For example, people with T-scores above the -2.5 cutoff generally have only 3 to 4 times greater risk than those below the cutoff, whereas differences in risk of 20 times are apparent when the full scale of BMD (or QUS) is used. Furthermore, fracture risk does not depend solely on BMD, but also on age and other risk factors, which should be taken into consideration. Many physicians are not familiar with this concept, and this is a major impediment to understanding and applying the results of risk assessment. One approach called remaining lifetime fracture probability (RLFP) calculates the risk of future fractures based on current BMD and age. The potential benefits of treatment to reduce bone loss rate can also be estimated (compared to an assumed average loss rate). At older ages, the reduced life expectancy limits the potential benefit of treatment.

A normogram is provided here for estimating RLFP (Fig. 29.1). In general, continuing treatment with estrogen (>5 years) or bisphosphonates (>2 years) will reduce fracture risk and the corresponding RLFP estimates by about half. Software to calculate RLFP is also available through at least one site on the Internet (www.medsurf.com). RLFP represents the average number of fractures during a patient's remaining life; patients with RLFP = 5 will experience an average of 5 fractures in the future. When risk is low (RLFP <1), patients will derive little benefit from treatment, because treatment cannot prevent many fractures. However, when RLFP is high, treatment can prevent multiple fractures.

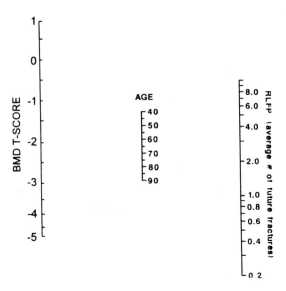

Figure 29.1. The T-score is calculated as the observed BMD minus the mean for women at age 35, divided by the standard deviation (SD) of BMD for young women. Thus, the T-score represents the number of SD above or below the mean BMD for young adult women. RLFP: remaining lifetime fracture probability.

Summary

Although osteoporosis affects the majority of elderly women and many men, only a small proportion of people have received risk assessment or treatment. To make wide-spread risk evaluation possible will require compact, fast, and inexpensive methods. Two likely candidates are quantitative ultrasound, and radiographic absorptiometry (or digital radiography). "User-friendly" statistical models such as remaining lifetime fracture probability will increase patient and physician acceptance and understanding of risk assessment. Better understanding, in turn, will help match high risk patients with more potent treatments, and reduce unnecessary treatment of low risk patients, as well as improving compliance.

Suggested Reading

Genant HK, Engelke K, Fuerst T et al. (1996) Noninvasive assessment of bone mineral and structure: state of the art. *J Bone Miner Res* 11: 707–730.

Ross PD, Wasnich RD, Davis JW. (1990) Fracture prediction models for osteoporosis prevention. *Bone* 11: 327–331.

30

Future Therapies

Ian R. Reid

At the present time, the therapy of osteoporosis is an intense focus of research for both commercial and non-commercial agencies. Some new therapies are likely to be introduced into clinical practice within the next 12 months, others are in phase 1–3 clinical trials, and still others have, to date, only been evaluated in the laboratory.

Bisphosphonates

The bisphosphonates (e.g. etidronate and alendronate) have recently become widely used in osteoporosis therapy. A number of new bisphosphonates of much greater anti-resorptive potency are under development. Their advent will result in the use of smaller doses and a probable reduction in gastrointestinal side-effects. The possibility of administering these agents by three monthly intravenous injections and by other non-oral routes, are also being studied. Current evidence suggests that more potent agents are unlikely to achieve greater increases in bone density than those already available, so these developments will contribute mainly to convenience and safety. Other means of interfering with osteoclast function are under investigation but it remains to be seen whether they will have any therapeutic advantages over the bisphosphonates.

Estrogen Agonists/Antagonists

The estrogen antagonist, tamoxifen, has partial estrogen-like effects on bone and lipid metabolism. These properties have led to interest in other agents of this class, which appear to have a variety of profiles of tissue-specific estrogen agonist/antagonist activities. Thus, tamoxifen acts as an agonist on lipid metabolism, bone and the endometrium, whereas it acts as an antagonist in the breast. Raloxifene, an agent now in phase 3 clinical trials, shares tamoxifen's agonist properties in bone and lipid metabolism, but is an anti-estrogen in both the endometrium and breast. This represents a very attractive range of activities, but the results of ongoing clinical studies will need to be awaited before their therapeutic potential can really be judged. The tissue-specific variability of agonist/antagonist properties of these compounds has led to the realization that the estrogen receptor and its regulation at the gene transcription level is much more complex than previously thought. This complexity is reflected in the new term for this class of compounds, selective estrogen receptor modulators

(SERMs). They are likely to play a major part in disease prevention in postmenopausal women, though their role in the management of established osteoporosis is less certain.

Bone Forming Agents

The real challenge in osteoporosis research has been to develop agents that stimulate bone formation, in contrast to estrogen-like compounds and bisphosphonates which are primarily anti-resorptives. Parathyroid hormone (PTH), growth hormone, and insulin-like growth factor 1 (IGF-1) are each the subject of current clinical trials. PTH, an 84-amino acid peptide, is one of the principal regulators of plasma calcium concentrations. It acts on bone via receptors on the osteoblast and stimulates both bone formation and resorption. Its effects on bone mass appear to depend upon the dose in which it is administered and the frequency of its administration. In general, intermittent treatment with low doses results in increased bone mass in animal studies. A number of analogues have now entered clinical trials, including PTH(1–34) and PTH(1–38), and analogues of the related peptide, parathyroid hormone-related protein. Several small clinical studies have showed substantial increases in density of trabecular bone, but there has been concern regarding the cortical bone loss in some studies. Co-administration with estrogen may overcome this problem.

Growth hormone acts directly on osteoblast-like cells causing the local production of IGF-1, which, in turn, acts as an autocrine regulator of osteoblast proliferation and protein synthesis. Growth hormone also regulates hepatic production of IGF-1 and the circulating levels of this protein may influence osteoblast activity. Growth hormone increases bone turnover (both formation and resorption) and reduces urinary calcium loss. There have been several trials of its use in humans over the last 30 years, most of which have not demonstrated clear-cut beneficial effects. As a result, it is not widely regarded as a promising therapy for osteoporosis. Attention has now moved to IGF-1, the administration of which increases bone turnover (both formation and resorption) in humans and causes fewer side-effects than growth hormone itself. Its effects on bone mass in clinical studies remain to be seen.

Other Agents Currently Under Investigation

There are many more potential therapies still being assessed in the laboratory, particularly other peptide growth factors. Transforming growth factor-β (TGF-β) and the bone morphogenic proteins (BMPs) belong to the same peptide family. They are produced by bone cells, are found in bone matrix, and probably have a role in the paracrine regulation of bone cell function, in particular promoting the growth of osteoblast precursors. Local or systemic administration of TGF-β *in vivo* stimulates bone formation. BMP2, platelet-derived growth factor, and megakaryocyte growth and differentiation factor are some of the other factors being similarly investigated. The future of any of these agents as a systemic therapy is open to some doubt because of their multiple target cells and consequent likelihood of significant non-bone effects.

Amylin is a 37-amino acid peptide co-secreted with insulin. It has recently been demonstrated that amylin and a number of related peptides have effects on osteoblast proliferation and bone mass *in vivo*, comparable to those of TGF-β. Analogues are being developed which retain the bone-active properties of this family of peptides but lack their other effects on carbohydrate metabolism and blood pressure. Research is also being conducted with non-peptide factors, including the zeolites (compounds made up of $(SiO_4)^{4-}$ and $(AlO_4)^{5-}$ tetrahedra) and strontium salts, which have been shown to promote osteoblast proliferation. These agents are all a long way from clinical use at present.

Summary

Research into novel therapies for osteoporosis is more active at present than at any time in the past. It has led to the recent use of the bisphosphonates in this area, and to the development of selective estrogen receptor modulators. Growth factors acting on osteoblasts are currently the focus of laboratory studies but much more work will be necessary before their probable clinical utility can be judged.

Suggested Reading

Cornish J, Callon KE, Cooper GJS, Reid IR. (1995) Amylin stimulates osteoblast proliferation and increases mineralized bone volume in adult mice. *Biochem Biophys Res Commun* 207: 133–139.

Grey AB, Stapleton JP, Evans MC, Tatnell MA, Ames RW, Reid IR. (1995) The effect of the antiestrogen tamoxifen on bone mineral density in normal late postmenopausal women. *Am J Med* 99: 636–641.

Holloway L, Butterfield G, Hintz RL, Gesundheit N, Marcus R. (1994) Effects of recombinant human growth hormone on metabolic indices, body composition, and bone turnover in healthy elderly women. *J Clin Endocrinol Metab* 79: 470–479.

Lindsay R, Cosman F, Nieves J, Dempster DW, Shen V. (1993) A controlled clinical trial of the effects of 1–34hPTH in estrogen treated osteoporotic women. *J Bone Miner Res* 8: s130.

Mundy GR. (1996) Regulation of bone formation by bone morphogenetic proteins and other growth factors. *Clin Orthop* 24–28.

Rudman D, Feller AG, Cohn L, Shetty KR, Rudman IW, Draper MW. (1991) Effects of human growth hormone on body composition in elderly men. *Horm Res* 36: Suppl 1: 73–81.

Yang NN, Venugopalan M, Hardikar S, Glasebrook A. (1996) Identification of an estrogen response element activated by metabolites of 17beta-estradiol and raloxifene. *Science* 273: 1222–1225.

31

How to Interpret New Data

Robert P. Heaney

"... experience is misleading, and judgement is difficult." – Hippocrates

A physician tries a new bone active agent in his practice; his patients seem to improve and he is enthusiastic. Another, trying the same agent, sees little patient improvement, but notes serious drug side effects, and becomes convinced that the drug is more trouble than it is worth. Both are wrong, as the Hippocratic maxim suggests. It is impossible to say how much of the difference between the two experiences is due to placebo effects, to variations in the biological makeup of the patients concerned, or simply to random chance.

General Study-design Considerations

Instead of relying solely upon personal experience with new diagnostic and treatment methods, a physician depends on studies reported in the medical literature. Such reports can be grouped into efficacy trials, studies of causation and risk, and cost-benefit analyses. While more reliable than anecdotal personal experience, these types of reports do not remove the need for judgement. Each type has distinct weaknesses as well as strengths.

Proof of efficacy of new agents is currently provided by double-blind, randomized, controlled trials (RCT), involving more than one medical center. Because this design eliminates the biases introduced both by the placebo effect and by the various selection factors which make one group of treated patients different from another, RCTs are now required by most national regulatory authorities for licensing of new drugs. Primary end points of these trials, applicable to the field of osteoporosis, will usually be bone mass or fracture rates. A useful agent will be one that reduces bone loss, leads to bone gain, or reduces fracture rate. The major strength of an RCT is that it permits strong causal inference, i.e., the conclusion that the differences found are really due to the test agent, rather than to other, unrecognized factors. Thus a positive result can be relied upon to mean that the drug is efficacious. The weakness of RCTs includes the fact that the design narrows the response range and thereby reduces the ability to find real effects that might be useful. Thus negative trials may mean little. Perhaps of more importance, many trials exclude subjects with a variety of co-morbid conditions and those taking other medications, i.e., precisely the kinds of situations commonly encountered in ordinary medical practice. Hence, while a positive RCT establishes that a drug is efficacious in its own right, it may tell a physician little about how the drug might act in his practice. It is also important to recall that many agents for which efficacy has not been established in an RCT, are not, *ipso facto*, ineffective. Many actually effective agents will never meet the standards of proof required in an RCT, because their target populations are too small, or the cost of studying them too high, or the available response range too limited.

Estimates of risk (or of causation) are mostly derived from observational or epidemiological studies, because using an RCT to expose people to possible harm is precluded on ethical grounds. Since observational studies do not permit strong causal inference, one must look for external supports for the purported causal relationship. Some helpful clues are: (1) consistency (similar findings in different studies); (2) proportionality (the risk rises with exposure); (3) sequence (the exposure precedes the effect); and (4) biological plausibility. It is also important to determine whether the finding arose from an *a priori* hypothesis or was the result of multiple comparisons performed to see what relationships might emerge. Most epidemiologic studies measure a sufficiently large number of variables that some are bound to be "significantly" correlated, just from random chance alone. Such outcomes are of dubious value.

Results of these kinds of studies are frequently reported as relative risks, or risk gradients, i.e., as estimates of the factor by which risk changes with exposure. A familiar example is the approximate doubling of fracture risk with every drop of one standard deviation in bone mineral density. But relative risk values, alone, give incomplete information. It is necessary also to know the *basal* risk of the outcome in question and to assess its importance, both medically and personally. Thus a regimen that increases endometrial cancer risk by the same 50% is of less importance than one that increases breast cancer risk by 50%. This is because basal risk of breast cancer is higher than that of endometrial cancer, and accordingly a 50% increase produces a larger number of cases than the same percent increase in endometrial cancer. Further, breast cancer is, overall, a more serious disorder, with a higher mortality. Finally, personal values enter into the judgement and influence the motivation to avoid risk. Thus, a regimen increasing breast cancer risk, but decreasing risk of myocardial infarction, will evoke different reactions in different women. Generally women fear breast cancer more than they fear coronary artery disease. There is no universally "correct" response in these circumstances.

The third major kind of report deals with cost-benefit analyses. These have become increasingly important in the development of practice guidelines, in the registration of drugs, and in the deployment of screening tests and preventive regimens. While it makes obviously good sense to practice medicine with greater rather than lesser efficiency, it is also true that, to some extent, all cost-benefit analyses are both arbitrary and based upon false premises. The purpose of medicine is not to reduce cost, but to reduce suffering, morbidity, and mortality. Doing so will always cost more than not doing so. Arbitrariness enters the equation in the judgement of how much is too much, as well as in how the costs and benefits are measured. In general it is much easier to calculate the costs of an intervention than to measure the savings it produces through disease prevention. Furthermore, there is a perverse element inherent in the use of cost-benefit analyses: as regulatory authorities escalate the standards of proof for a new drug, the cost of meeting those standards rises, and the price of the drug increases in parallel, thus negatively affecting the cost benefit profile of the drug.

Special Skeletal Considerations

The results of treatment trials of bone active agents must be analyzed in a way consistent with the underlying biology. In general, that means that early period responses must be analyzed separately from later responses. This is because osteoporotic fragility is the result of many years of bone loss and/or structural deterioration, because bone mass changes very slowly, and because the bone remodeling processes of formation and resorption are asynchronous.

If the primary outcome variable is fracture, and if the agent being tested acts through an effect on bone mass, then it should be obvious that fractures occurring soon after starting treatment will reflect *pre*-treatment fragility, and not the effect of the treatment *per se*. Later on (after at least one year), when the treatment has had a chance to affect bone mass appreciably, the real effect of the agent, if any, will be manifest. By contrast, an agent affecting central nervous system reflexes, and thereby reducing falls in the elderly, would be expected to have an immediate effect, which could be tested much sooner.

Somewhere from 2 to 20% of the skeleton may be involved in remodeling at any given time, and because remodeling loci are largely demineralized, this bony component is not detected by densitometry. Remodeling suppressive agents, such as calcitonin and the bisphosphonates, reduce the size of this "remodeling space", and over the several month remodeling life cycle, they reclaim a portion of that previously remodeling bone. This increase in bone mass is called a "remodeling transient". But it is not actually *new* bone; nor does this change predict the effect of the agent on bone balance. This distinction is shown in Figure 31.1. Line A represents the time course of bone density in the untreated state. Lines B–D show

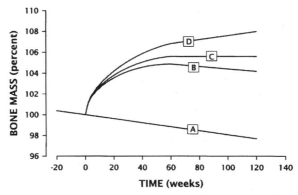

Figure 31.1. Time course of changes in bone mass in different clinical situations. A = untreated, B–D = treated. See text for explanations.

the effects of three remodeling suppressors. All produce a transient amounting to about a 5% gain in bone mass, fully expressed at about one year. But agent B fails to alter remodeling balance, and bone loss continues as before, although from a higher baseline. Agent C, by contrast, stops bone loss entirely, and agent D actually leads to slight bone gain. Only by analyzing the data after one year can the three patterns be distinguished.

Surprisingly, many osteoporosis trials fail to give adequate consideration to these features unique to the response of bone, and their reports often combine (and confuse) the early and late phase results. Thus, despite the trend toward greater evidential rigor, experience remains misleading, and judgement is no less difficult.

Suggested Reading

Heaney RP. (1996) Design considerations for osteoporosis trials. In: Marcus R, Feldman D, Kelsey J (eds) *Osteoporosis*. Academic Press, San Diego pp. 1125–1142.

32

Socio-economic Impact

L. Joseph Melton III

Osteoporotic fractures pose an enormous public health problem, and a variety of interventions will be needed to reduce their impact. The only rationale for risk assessment is to employ these interventions efficiently. However, screening tests have costs and the long-term benefits of treatment may be uncertain. This creates a need to consider the costs of risk assessment and the costs of treatment as well as the costs of fractures that might be averted.

Costs of Osteoporosis

Fractures are ubiquitous. The lifetime risk of one or more of them in a 50-year-old white woman is 75%. Even considering only the fractures traditionally associated with osteoporosis (hip, spine and distal forearm), the lifetime risk is about 40% and, in a 50-year-old white man, 13%. These fractures lead to a considerable burden of disability and cost. Thus, it has been estimated that white women aged 45 years or over in the United States will experience 5.2 million fractures of the hip, spine or distal forearm over the next ten years, leading to 2 million person-years of fracture-related disabilities and to over US$45 billion in direct medical expenditures. The greatest amount of disability and cost is attributable to hip fractures, and other analyses concur that hip fracture is far and away the most important complication of osteoporosis by almost any measure. However, all of these fractures are associated with serious reductions in patient function and quality of life.

The cost of managing the large number of fractures that occur each year is great. Direct medical expenditures for osteoporotic fractures in the United States in 1995 have been estimated at US$13.8 billion. Charges for hospitalization (US$8.6 billion) and nursing home care (US$3.9 billion) were the major contributors to overall cost, which was dominated by expenditures for the care of hip fractures (over US$30,000 per episode). Costs will rise dramatically in the future with growth of the elderly population. In Europe, persons age 65 years and over are expected to increase from about 68 million in 1990 to over 133 million in 2050, with a corresponding 80% increase in the annual number of hip fractures. If hip fracture incidence rates continue to increase as they have in many countries, the number of fractures and their associated costs will be greater still.

Costs of Risk Assessment

With a public health approach to osteoporosis control, interventions are applied to everyone in order to improve some characteristic (e.g. bone density) in the population as a whole. No individual risk assessment is needed and costs relate solely to the interventions (see below). The clinical approach of early detection and treatment of high-risk individuals, on the other hand, often requires screening. Risk assessments might be aimed at low bone mineral density, excessive bone turnover or an increased likelihood of falling. Elevated bone turnover is common in elderly women and is an independent risk factor for fractures. If pharmacologic agents were deployed specifically to manipulate bone formation or resorption, biochemical markers of bone turnover would be needed to identify appropriate patients for treatment. No testing or treating algorithm has been developed, however, so it is not possible to estimate the cost of this approach. Similarly, development of multifaceted programs to prevent falls or to alter the biomechanical consequences of a fall (e.g. energy absorbing hip pads) will require screening for a high likelihood of falling. No cost estimates are available for this activity either.

Most analyses have focused on mass screening for low bone density. Unselective screening of every woman at menopause would be quite expensive. Moreover, at a cost of US$53,610 per life year saved, an analysis by the Office of Technology Assessment indicates that it is not cost-effective to screen 50 year-old white women with dual energy x-ray absorptiometry of the hip in order to treat those more than 1 SD below the mean (about 16% of the population) with hormone replacement therapy (HRT) for 20 years. More hip fractures would be prevented by widespread use of HRT and, although costs would be higher, the cost per life year saved would be less (Table 32.1). Cost-effectiveness would also improve with longer treatment since most adverse events prevented by HRT occur late in life. However, the analysis was dominated by extraskeletal effects of HRT. Thus, the cost per year of life saved might increase from US$23,334 for universal HRT treatment for 40 years to US$43,765 if a decade of HRT doubled the risk of breast cancer instead of raising it by 35% as was assumed. Conversely, the cost per life year saved might fall to US$7,153 if the risk of myocardial infarction while on HRT were reduced by 80% instead of 50%. Most other analyses have reached the same general conclusions.

However, an extensive analysis by the National Osteoporosis Foundation shows that selective screening with bone densitometry is cost-effective among women at high risk of fracture on the basis of low bone density, risk factors (family history of fractures, low body weight and cigarette smoking) or a personal history of fracture. This is particularly important with respect to drugs whose beneficial effects are limited to the skeleton. The Office of Technology Assessment estimated that initiating therapy at age 50 with such a drug at a cost of US$1,000 per year would imply a cost per life year saved of nearly US$750,000 if all women were treated and over US$360,000 even if treatment were limited to women with osteopenia. Other analyses agree that unselective use of relatively expensive drugs is unlikely to be cost-effective, especially if the treatments, themselves, have any adverse influence on quality of life.

Table 32.1. Lifetime hip fracture risk (%) and cost per life year saved (US$) under different strategies for screening 50 year-old women for bone mineral density (BMD) and using estrogen replacement therapy (ERT).

Duration of ERT	Screen, BMD threshold			
	No screening, no ERT	Screen, ERT for BMD < −1 SD	Screen, ERT for BMD < mean	No screening, all on ERT
No ERT				
Fracture risk	17.0	−	−	−
Cost	Baseline	−	−	−
10 years				
Fracture risk	−	16.0	14.4	12.9
Cost	−	US$151,392	US$134,644	US$126,876
20 years				
Fracture risk	−	15.3	12.4	9.8
Cost	−	US$53,610	US$42,724	US$45,761
30 years				
Fracture risk	−	14.8	11.2	7.8
Cost	−	US$28,257	US$29,357	US$31,059
40 years				
Fracture risk	−	14.7	10.9	7.2
Cost	−	US$27,486	US$22,431	US$23,334

(Modified from U.S. Congress, Office of Technology Assessment (1995) Appendix C: Evidence on HRT and bone loss. In: *Effectiveness and Costs of Osteoporosis Screening and Hormone Replacement Therapy, Volume II: Evidence on Benefits, Risks, and Costs.* OTA-BP-H-144,. U.S. Government Printing Office, Washington, DC pp 19–33.)

Costs of Treatment

Due to the very large size of the affected population, the cost of treatment is a major issue. If interventions are cheap and safe enough (some forms of calcium and vitamin D), they may be employed indiscriminately as a public health measure. This can be done without risk assessment, although screening may be cost-effective if more expensive forms of calcium and vitamin D are used. Public health approaches will also be needed to promote maximum peak bone mass through improved diet and exercise, although few such programs exist and there are no estimates of cost on a population basis. The Office of Technology Assessment concluded that almost ten times more life years would be saved by universal HRT at the menopause, compared to targeting such therapy to women with low bone density, if estrogen actually reduces the risk of heart disease. However, the cost of treating every woman in the United States age 50 years or over with HRT, even at US$258–269 per year, could exceed the annual cost of hip fractures. Bone-specific agents (e.g. bisphosphonates, calcitonin) are not likely to be used so widely, and their cost (and cost-effectiveness) depends upon who is treated. This remains controversial.

Summary

Osteoporotic fractures exact a dreadful toll of pain, disability and expense. Because virtually the entire population is at risk for osteoporosis, inexpensive public health approaches are needed to help prevent the condition but they are not well developed. Pharmacological treatment of the entire population would be prohibitively expensive so risk assessment is needed to employ costly drugs more efficiently. Screening itself may be expensive, however, and efforts continue to define cost-effective approaches to the identification and treatment of individual patients at high risk for osteoporotic fractures.

Suggested Reading

Chrischilles E, Shireman T, Wallace R. (1994) Costs and health effects of osteoporotic fractures. *Bone* 15: 377–386.

Eddy D, Cummings SR, Dawson-Hughes B, Johnston CC, Lindsay R, Melton LJ III, Slemenda C. (in press) Guidelines for the prevention, diagnosis and treatment of osteoporosis: Cost-effectiveness analysis and review of the evidence. *Osteoporosis Int.*

Greendale GA, Barrett-Connor E, Ingles S, Haile R. (1995) Late physical and functional effects of osteoporotic fracture in women: The Rancho Bernardo Study. *J Am Geriatr Soc* 43: 955–961.

Ray NF, Chan JK, Thamer M, Melton LJ III. (1997) Medical expenditures for the treatment of osteoporotic fractures in the United States in 1995: Report from the National Osteoporosis Foundation. *J Bone Miner Res* 12: 24–35.

Torgerson DJ, Kanis JA. (1995) Cost-effectiveness of preventing hip fractures in the elderly population using vitamin D and calcium. *Q J Med* 88: 135–139.

U.S. Congress, Office of Technology Assessment. (1995) *Effectiveness and Costs of Osteoporosis Screening and Hormone Replacement Therapy. Volume I: Cost-Effectiveness Analysis*, OTA-BP-H-160. U.S. Government Printing Office, Washington, DC.

U.S. Congress, Office of Technology Assessment. (1995) *Effectiveness and Costs of Osteoporosis Screening and Hormone Replacement Therapy. Volume II: Evidence on Benefits, Risks, and Costs*. OTA-BP-H-144. U.S. Government Printing Office, Washington, DC.

Index